Complete Book of Yoga

Published by :
Lotus Press Publishers & Distributors

Complete Book of Yoga

Dr. Deepika M. Sharma
M.B.B.S. P.G. D.H.H.
and
Dr. Rajeev Sharma
MD., D. Lit

Lotus PRESS
4735/22, Prakash Deep Building
Ansari Road, Darya Ganj,
New Delhi - 110002

Lotus Press : Publishers & Distributors
Unit No. 220, 2nd Floor, 4735/22, Prakash Deep Building,
Ansari Road, Darya Ganj, New Delhi- 110002
Ph.: 41325510, 98118-38000
• E-mail : lotuspress1984@gmail.com
www.lotuspress.co.in

Complete Book of Yoga

ISBN: 81-8382-196-0

Printed & Published by : **Lotus Press Publishers & Distributors,** New Delhi-02

Preface

It gives me immense pleasure to write this book. Yoga is the union of this physical body to mind then mind to soul and then soul to the Universe.To achieve this peak, where one can unite with the universe–the yoga is one of the great steps.

Here in this book I have tried to write in simple language so that the common man can understand the methods and can be benefitted. Besides regular yogic exercises, I have included the simple exercises also which can be practised any time like laughing, palming, accu-massage etc.

I have included the shat-karma, tratak, meditation, different important yogic exercises etc; besides the simple ones. Exercises for children like tarasana, exercises for gastric problems like pavanmuktasana, exersises to reduce belly and obesity like paschimottanasana, exercises for proper energy flow and exercises for relaxation like shavasana are well described along with colour photographs,respectively.

I am thankful to Dr.Deepika M. Sharma for co-authoring this book.

I am highly thankful to Ms.Aishrwaya, Ms.Aditi, Ms.Medhavi and Mr.Tejaswi for giving nice poses for different yogasanas.

I am thankful to my wife Jyoti for cooperating in completion of this project.

Hope readers will find it useful.

With thanks and regards,

Dr.Rajeev Sharma

Contents

Preface

1. It's Your Body **01-20**

- The Bones 1
- The Muscles 2
- The Circulation 2
- The Nerves 4
- The Reproduction 4
- Male Organs 9
- Female Organs 14

2. Some Important Points Before Starting Yogic Exercises **21-26**

- Yoga and Food 21
- Yoga and Mind 22
- Yoga and Pranayama 22
- Multiple Benefits of Yoga 23
- Importance of Yogic Exercises 25
- Precautions 25

3.	**Factors Necessary for Performance of Yogasanas**	**27-30**
	• Time	27
	• Place	28
	• Rest	28
	• Bath	29
	• Dress	29
	• Breakfast	29
	• Sunbath	29
	• General	30
4.	**Asanas and Diseases (Disorders)**	**31-34**
5.	**Root Cause of All Problems–Energy Imbalance**	**35-44**
	• Physical Factors	35
	• Mental Factors	36
	• Imbalance Towards Left Side	40
	• Imbalance Towards Right Side	41
	• Balance at the Centre	41
	• Balance of Nadis	42
	• Clearing the Chakras	42
6.	**Important Yogasanas for Everyone**	**45-57**
	• Padmasana	45
	• Vajrasana	46
	• Bhujangasana	46
	• Gomukhasana	47
	• Sarvangasana	48

- Chakrasana 49
- Kagasana 49
- Kukkutasana 50
- Mahavirasana 50
- Mayurasana 51
- Parvatasana 52
- Yanasana 52
- Matsyasana 53
- Paschimottanasana 54
- Janushirasana 54
- Ushtrasana 55
- Sinhmudra 55
- Mandukasana 56

7. Asanas to Reduce Obesity, Diabetes, Thyroid and Other Disorders 58-59

- Trikonasana 58
- Padhastasana 58
- Shashankasana 58
- Ushtrasana 59
- Yoganidra 59
- Tratak 59

8. Asanas to Increase Height, Stretch Spine, Eye Exercises, Control Digestive System, Hasya Yoga, Accupressure and Others 60-62

- Sarvottanasana 60
- Butterfly 61
- Accupressure Exercises 61

- Hasya Yoga 61
- Spinal Stretch 61
- Height Increasing Poses (Tarasana and Vrikshasana) 62
- Eye exercises 62

9. Mudras for Quick Relief 63-68

- Gyan Mudra 63
- Vairagya Mudra 64
- Abhay Mudra 64
- Dhyan Mudra 64
- Vayuu Mudra 65
- Shoonya Mudra 65
- Surya Mudra 65
- Varun Mudra 66
- Prithvi Mudra 66
- Prana Mudra 66
- Apaan Mudra 67

10. Shat-Karma–The Cleansing Exercises 69-77

- Dhauti 69
- Basti 70
- Neti 71
- Tratak 74
- Nauli 75
- Kapalbhati 76
- Agnisar 77

11. Surya Namaskar–Ek Chamatkar 78-81

12. Powerful Yogic Exercises–Bandha (Locks) 82-85

- Jalandhar Bandha 82
- Mula Bandha 83
- Uddiyan Bandha 84
- Master Lock 84

13. Breathing Process and Elements of Prana 86-95

- The Lungs 88
- The Ribcage 89
- The Diaphragm 89
- Breath Volumes 90
- Nose and its Utility 91
- The Respiratory System 92
- The Theory of Relaxation and Breathing 93
- Abdominal Breathing 93
- How Oxygen Reaches the Blood Stream 94
- Physiological Effects of Stress and Relaxation 94

14. Panchkarma–Sub Divisions of Prana 96-97

- Pran Vayu 96
- Udan Vayu 96
- Samana Vayu 96
- Apana Vayu 97
- Vyana Vayu 97

15. Scientific Way of Breathing 98-101

16. Some Important Guidelines for Pranayama 102-104

- Abdominal breathing 103
- Chest breathing 104

- Yogic breathing 104

17. Pranayama–The Methods and Meaning **105-108**

- Methods of Pranayama 105
- Rhythmic Respiration 106
- Variations in Rhythmic Breathing Process 106
- Kriyas during Pranayama 107

18. Pranayama–It's Healing Powers and Benefits **109-116**

- Procedure of Pranayama 109
- The Two Naris 110
- Benefits of Pranayama 110
- Kinds of Pranayama 111
  1. Surya Bhedan 111
  2. Ujjai 112
  3. Sitkari 112
  4. Shitali 113
  5. Bhastrika 113
  6. Brahmari 114
  7 Moorcha 114
  8 Plavini 115
  9 Breathing 115
  10.Exercises 115

19. Science of Chanting–Japa Yoga **117-121**

- Rules for Chanting of Mantras 119
- Ajapa-Japa 120
- Precautions and Guidelines 121

20. **Aura–A Luminous Cloud** 122-124

21. **Inner Visualization–Antah Darshan** 125-131

- Cidkasa darsana 126
- Antarmauna 126
- Yogic and Tantric Dharna 130
- Udanisadic Dharna 131

22. **Meditation–The Scientific Way** 132-141

- Concentration 132
- Dainandini Dhyana 135
- Vigara Dhyana 135
- Mantra Dhyana 135
- Svasa Dhyana 136
- Sahaja Dhyana 137
- Nada Dhyana 137
- Bhava Dhyana 139
- Unmani Kriya 140

23. **Science of Vital Energy (Prana-Vidya)** 142-147

- Procedure 143
- Kundali Vidya 144
- Important facts related to Meditation 145

24. **Chakras–The Source of Energy** 148-155

- Chakras-Spinning Energy Wheels 148
- Chakra Colours and Key Words 151
- The Cleansing Breath Technique 153
- Nadi Sadhana 153
- Chakra Chart II 154

25. Yogic Exercises for Relaxation	**156-162**
• Shavasana	156
• Makrasana	160
• Balasana	161
26. Diet for the Yoga Practitioners	**163-168**
• Acid Producing Foods	166
• Alkali Producing Foods	166
• Foods to be Replaced	166
• Ideal Menu and Timing	167
27. Nature's Tonic–Drink Water in Early Morning	**169-172**
28. Tips with Yoga	**173-177**

1.
IT'S YOUR BODY

Before starting yoga one should know about human body and its functioning.

There are eight basic systems of the human body (i) Bones (ii) Muscles (iii) Circulation (iv) Nerves (v) Respiration (vi) Digestion (vii) Excretion and (viii) Reproduction. We shall discuss these one by one.

The Bones

The bony skeleton supporting the human body is constructed to strengthen the muscles which produce movement in the body to give shape. The forelimbs of the human body are supported by bones forming a shoulder girdle and similarly the leg bones are connected to others forming a pelvic girdle. Ribs connected to the backbone (including those connected to the breast bone) serve to protect certain internal organs, including the heart and the lungs. Man's structural superiority over other animals is due to the straight femur or thigh bone and the erect poise of the head.

The above features enable the man to walk in an erect position so that his hands are there to perform other functions. These structural advantages and the formation of his skull and lower jaw are responsible for an increase in brain power and intelligence in man, as compared with the other animals.

The human system consists of 206 bones of various sizes. The bones are composed of cells, which are softer in early childhood than in adult life. Where bones meet there is a joint which may simply be an immovable joint as in the bones of the skull or may be movable joint as that of the knee. The movable joints are necessary for the motion of human body.

The Muscles

Muscles are attached to the bones and consist of bundles of fleshly fibres, capable of contraction or shortening. When required such contractions help the various limbs of the body to move. The muscles are of two kinds namely the voluntary muscles whose movements are controlled by human will and the involuntary muscles which perform their function without any conscious effort of the will. These include the heart, the muscles of the stomach and those of the intestines. Their movements are rhythmic and we are not conscious of their action.

The Circulation

This system comprises the blood and heart and their functions. The blood is continuously propelled by the contraction of the heart and is derived into the arteries. The arteries are elastic tubes which by their recoil aid the distribution of the blood to all parts.

The blood is a clear fluid comprising innumberable solid bodies called corpuscles. The corpuscles are of two kinds–red and white–and are cellular shaped. The red corpuscles carry haemoglobin which constitutes protein and a little iron.

When combined with oxygen haemoglobin forms a bright red substance. The white corpuscles are living organisms, small jelly like creatures each with a nucleus. They are of great importance as they eat up the disease germs that enter the body. They are capable of independent movement in the blood stream and within the tissue and can swallow up dead bacteria and foreign particles.

HUMAN BODY

ORGANS

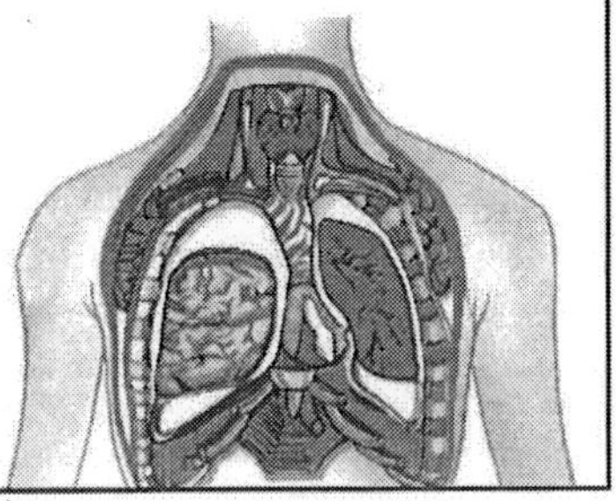

CRANIAL

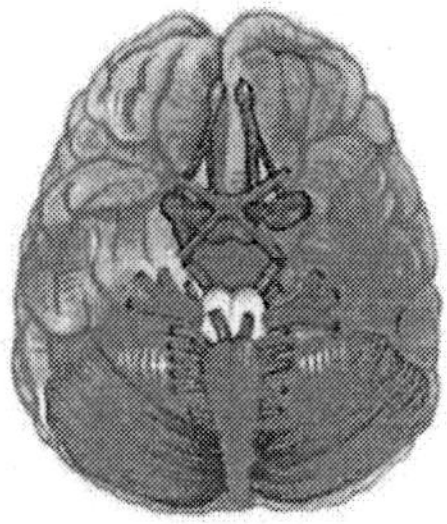

EYE

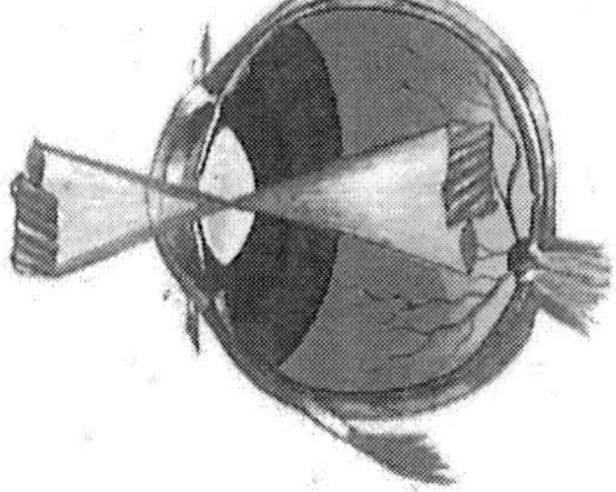

EAR

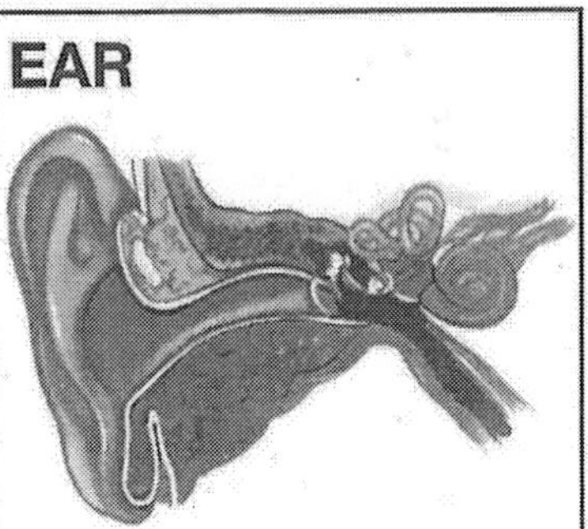

NOSE

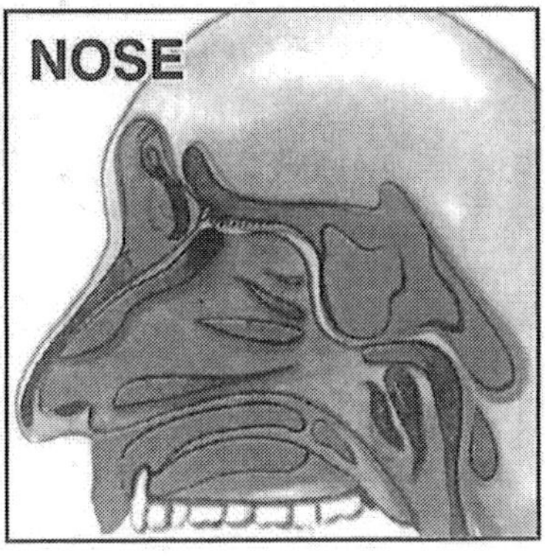

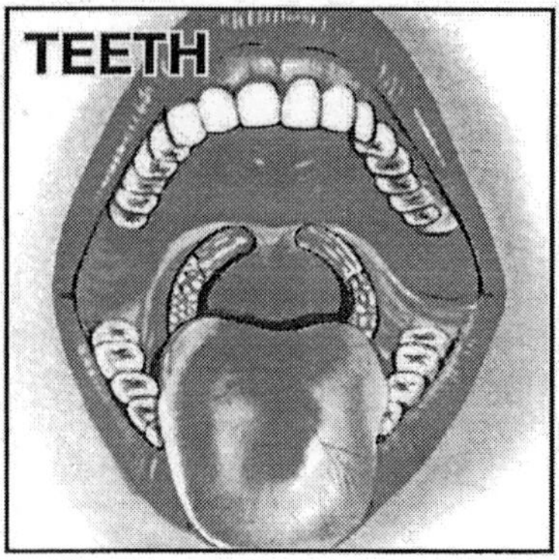
TEETH

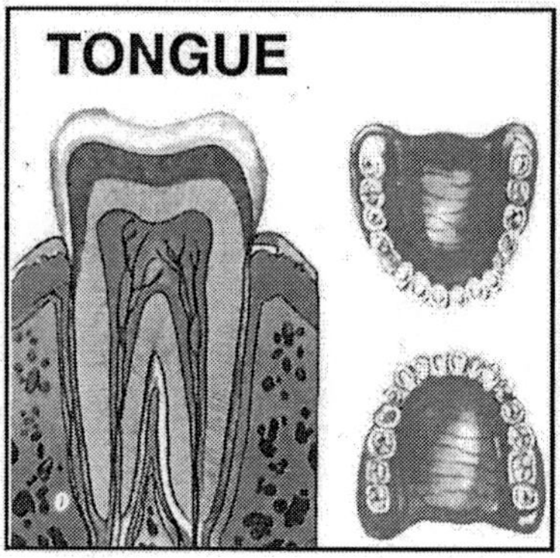
TONGUE

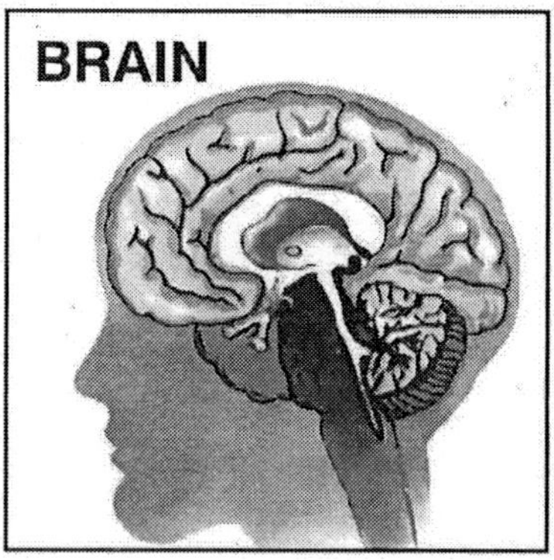
BRAIN

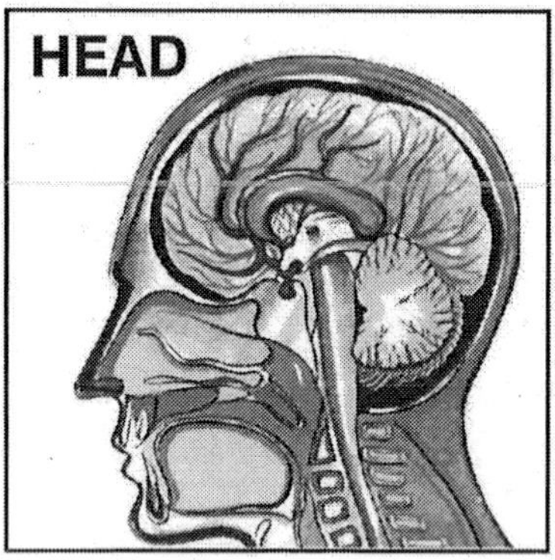
HEAD

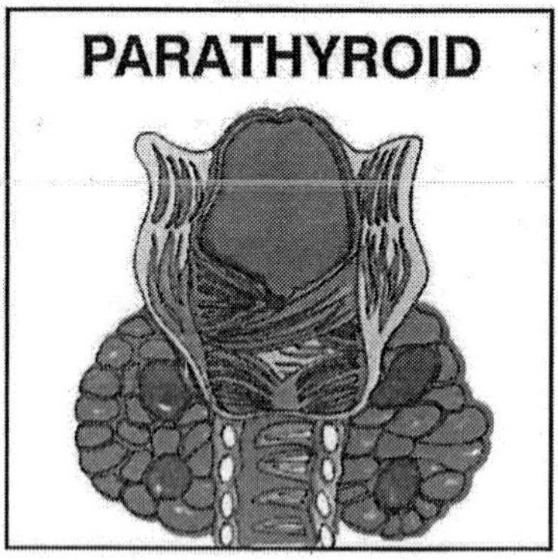
PARATHYROID

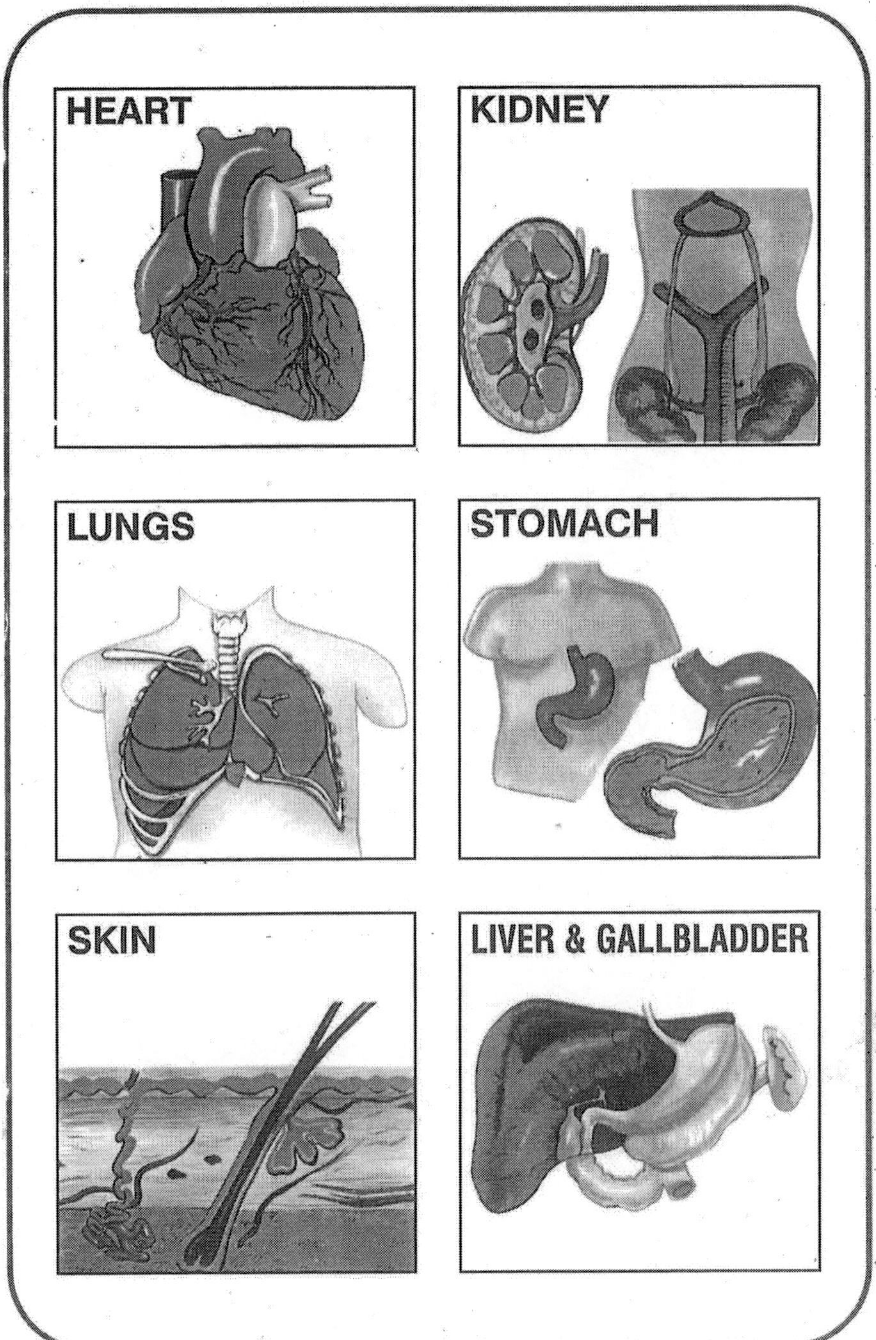
HEART
KIDNEY
LUNGS
STOMACH
SKIN
LIVER & GALLBLADDER

BLOOD CIRCULATION

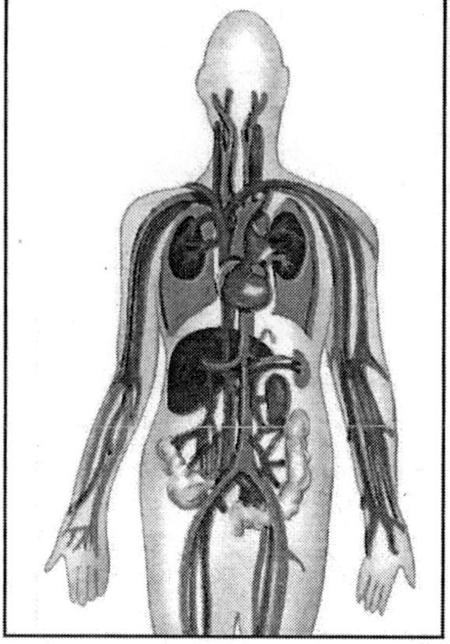

SKELETON

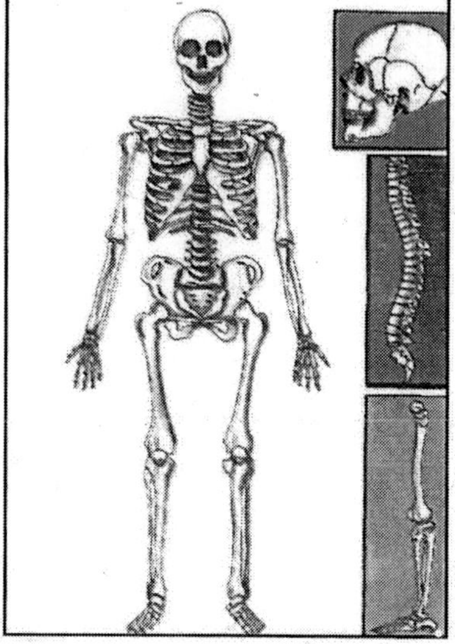

DIGESTIVE SYSTEM

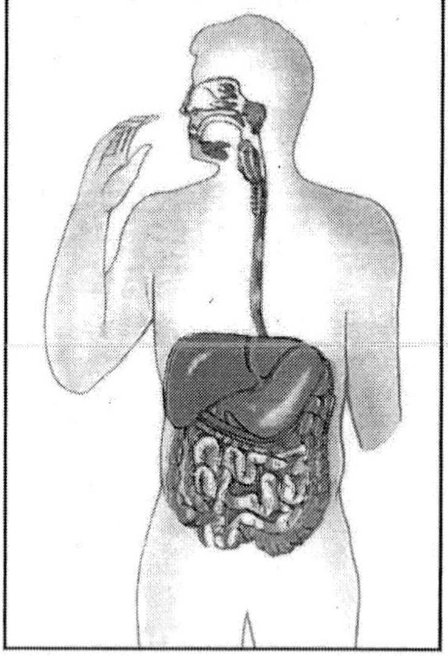

MUSCLES

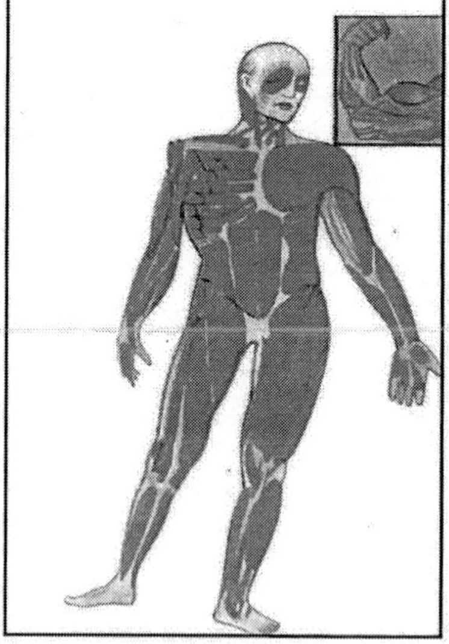

The main functions of blood are the following:

- It carries oxygen to every part of the body that requires it.
- It carries impurities from all parts of the body to the excretory organs namely the lungs, the kidneys and the skin.
- It carries food from the digestive system to all tissues.
- It carries heat to all parts of the body.

The heart is a hollow, muscular and somewhat conical four chambered force pump enclosed in a fibrous bag. It is situated in the chest between the lungs and weigh from 10 to 12 ounces. The heart is divided into two parts by a wall running from top to bottom with no direct connection between the parts. These parts are themselves divided into parts, upper and lower but have valves between them. The upper portions are called Auricles and the lower ones Ventricles.

When the blood reaches the tissues it loses all its oxygen and is loaded with waste materials especially carbon dioxide from the tissues. The impure blood reaches the heart by means of capillaries and veins. With the beat of the heart, it enters into the Right Auricle and then to the Right Ventricle from where it is taken by the Pulmonary Artery to the lungs. In the lungs capillaries, the blood comes into contact with oxygen and is purified (oxygenated). The purified blood is now brought back to heart by means of Pulmonary Vein. It now enters the left Auricle and when Auricles are contracted during the heart beat, the blood passes to the left Ventricle and then commences its journey again to all parts of the body. Thus with the contraction of right and left auricles, the venous blood from the body and aerated (oxygenated) blood from the lungs is pumped into their respective ventricles. And when the right and left ventricles contract, venous blood is pumped into the lungs and the aerated blood into the main vessels. These rhythmic contractions and dilations followed by an equivalent pause are called pulse or heart beat.

The Nerves

It is the most important system as it commands rest of the body what to do and how to work together. While the central nervous system resides in the skull and the spine, the nerves are spread all over the body. The nervous system of a man is a network pervading the whole body, having two way connection with the central control and enabling the individual to give a coordinated response to any stimulus from outside. Thus nerves that carry the messages to the muscles with orders to perform a particular action are called Motor Nerves.

The brain is the chief centre of the nervous system and is contained within the skull. The brain susbstance consists of grey and white matter. The grey matter forming a thin, superficial layer (cortex). It consists of three parts: (a) the cerebrum or bigger brain, which governs our consciousness, thought, emotions, will, sight, hearing, sensation of pain and memory through the grey matter, (b) the cerebellum or the smaller brain is connected with the coordination of the actions, nervous and muscular, by which the movement of the body are carried on, (c) Medulla Oblongata houses the centre of nervous tissue connected with reflex action consisting of movements that take place automatically, such as breathing or walking.

The spinal cord consist mostly of nerves. This is like a continuation of the medulla and runs down the back, surrounded by the bony arch of the spinal column. This organ is capable of making simple decisions, called the reflex action.

The Respiration

This system comprises lungs and the passages leading to them.

The purpose of respiration (breathing) is the entry and exit of air to and from the lungs. The object of breathing is to bring oxygen of the air into contact with the blood with the purpose of (a) giving some oxygen to the blood and (b) taking out waste products from the blood.

The air, in going to the lungs, has to go through various passages. They are nose or mouth, and the larynx or voice box.

We breathe through nose or through mouth. There are two passages leading downwards from nose and mouth into the body. One takes food and water to the stomach and the other takes air to the lungs.

Larynx or voice box is commonly known as "Adam's Apple" and can easily be felt in the throat. It is a cavity (in throat) holding vocal cords. Vibration of cords produces vocal sounds. The air passes from the voice box to the lungs by means of wind pipe which is about four inches long and one inch wide. The wind pipe at the lower end, is divided into two branches that go to the lungs.

The functioning of the lungs has already been described while discussing the Excretory System. The functioning of lungs as the respiratory organ is slightly more complicated. In the lungs, the air gets very close to the blood, that comes from the whole body through heart. The impure blood, dark red in colour, has too much carbon dioxide in it. This blood comes from the tissues, which have taken the oxygen from it but have loaded it with carbon dioxide. In the tissues, oxygen is used every minute to burn up the food material, resulting in production of considerable quantity of carbon dioxide. The lung's function is to reverse this state of affairs, i.e. restoring its oxygen quota and expelling the excess carbon dioxide. Thus the venous blood (the impure blood) is rendered arterial (bright red in colour) in its passage through the lung capillaries. It goes back to the heart and is ready to do its work again. The fresh oxygen, taken by the blood all over the body, is picked up again by its muscles which need it for their normal functioning.

The Digestion

The food that we take comprises proteins, sugars and starches, vitamins, salts, fats and oils. Only a part of these substances is useful to the body and the rest, which is indigestible, must be get rid of. The food is broken up by the teeth and after getting mixed with saliva, it is swallowed. Saliva is an alkaline fluid which is also common to the air passage at this level. It then passes into the gullet. Like stomach and intestines, the gullet is a muscular organ and can force the food along if necessary. With the help of the muscle, a man can drink even if he is standing on his head. About nine inches long, the gullet ends in the stomach. It is here that the second stage of digestion takes place.

From this position the food reaches stomach which is a hollow muscular organ lined by a glandular mucus membrane which secretes the gastric juice containing hydrochloric acid, salts, pepsin and water. The stomach mixes the food well by moving it round and round. At one stage the proteins are changed to a form in which they can pass through the stomach well and be absorbed, at once, ready to nourish the body.

Starches and proteins are now acted upon, though not digested completely. Fat and oil are broken up and oil is set free. In the stomach, digestion may take two to three hours. The food then goes to small intestine which is a long tube which, when uncoiled, may measure about one feet. Here, we have to consider the action of three different digestive juices, e.g., the pancreatic juice, the bile generated by the liver and the intestinal juice, which is the secretion of the small glands of the bowel lining. Food passes through the intestine and finally nutrients are absorbed and carried into the blood. The bile and the pancreatic juices are produced by the liver and pancreas respectively.

Liver is the largest organ in the body, which is situated just underneath the diaphragm rather on the right side. Its weight is about three to four pounds. There are fine tubes in the liver called bile ducts into which the cells of the liver secrets bile, and the bile ducts join together and form hepatic duct which carries the bile to the duodenum (also known as first part of small intestine).

Bile is a yellow fluid, containing mucus, water and some salts (called bile salts). It acts on the fats and oils and breaks them up into very small particles.

Liver is also a storehouse for sugar which it puts in the blood, when it is required by the body. About seven inches long, there is another large gland reddish in colour and known as Pancreas. It lies behind the stomach, and tube from it called the Pancreatic duct enters the intestine near where the bile duct enters. The pancreatic juices act on the protein, the starches and the fats.

The intestine is an organ of digestion as well as of absorption. The food, now digested, can pass through the walls of the intestine and is taken into the blood. It is then distributed all over the body. Food remains in the small intestine for about 12 hours and is slowly passed on towards the large intestine.

The large intestine is a 6 feet long tube. It is little concerned with the digestion or absorption of food, for more of this has already been done. Food remains here from 24 to 36 hours. Due to loss of water, the material in the large intestine now hardens as it reaches the rectum. Finally, the ingestible remnant is turned out.

The Excretion

It comprises the kidney, skin, lungs and bowels. The system is designed to help get rid of the waste matter in the body when all juices have been extracted from the digestive food. There are two kidneys, situated one on each side of the backbone in the small portion of the back or loin. It has the renal artery which brings blood to it and the renal vein which takes it away. In addition, there are the usual nerves, the lymphatic vessels and the ureter, the tube that takes urine from the kidney to the bladder which is the reservoir for urine.

Urine, a pale yellow fluid, carrying the waste nitrogen from our protein foods, and also mineral salts, secreted into the two kidneys. The kidney may be regarded as a pair of filters, through which about 2 pints of blood circulates every minute. In fact, the whole blood in the body passes down to the kidneys in five to six minutes. Urine is propelled down along the ureters from the kidneys to the bladder by successive veins of contraction in the muscular walls of these channels.

The bladder is an elastic membrane serving as temporary reservoir for urine, secreted by the kidneys. The normal adult capacity is about 1 pint. The urine is discharged into the bladder in intermittent jets every 20 seconds or so. The outlet below the bladder is normally closed by a tight ring of muscle called sphincter. In emptying, the bladder contracts and the sphincter relaxes to allow efflux of urine.

Another important agent for excretion of the waste material from the body is skin. It has two layers, the top one called the epidermis and dermis or true skin below the epidermis.

The latter is richly supplied with blood vessels. The skin is designed to:

- protect the body;
- acts as an organ of excretion by means of sweat glands. It thus helps to regulate the temperature of the body and;
- to give the sense of touch.

The skin has hair and sense organs. The latter are little lumps in the dermis which are nerve endings. They report to the nervous system when anything comes into their contant. The skin also has two kinds of glands, the Sebaceous glands, which secrete an oily substance serving as lubricant to the skin and the Sweat glands which make the skin as an excretory organ. The function of the latter is to take up sweat from the blood and pour it out on the skin. Though mostly water, the sweat contains, salts, fats and tiny bits of skin.

Bowels are the intestines, both large and small, which serve to complete the digestion of food and to allow its absorption into the blood stream. The useless or undigested food remains are gradually moved onwards and are hardened in the large intestine wherefrom they are ready to be thrown out. The failure of the bowel function is called constipation.

Lumps comprise two elastic spongy masses, almost filling the chest cavity. These are important agents to cleanse the system of impurity. Lungs throw off carbon dioxide, water (in the shape of vapour) and also some organic matter.

They are, therefore, organs of excretion in addition to being the organs of respiration

The Reproduction

Reproductive organs play an important role as chakras and hormonal secretion is directly associated with this system. Here is the description of these organs-

Male Organs

The sex organs of a male are quite complicated form of a reproductive system. They produce semen stored it and release into the woman's vagina at the time of ejaculation. Procreation, therefore, is the result of the union of the sperm cell and the ovum.

Testes

The male organs comprise of the two testes of testicles hung side by side in a sac called the scrotum, behind the penis in its relaxed state. The testes are oval in shape and about an inch long and inch wide, have two different functions. These are made up of a series of lobes composed of minute tubules in which the sperm cells the spermatozoa are formed and liberated. The internal secretion of sex hormones which create sex impulses and cause the essential male characteristics in the individual and play its role with the other secretory glands in the body in sustaining the normal functioning of the body, are achieved by it. In case this function is impaired before puberty, the development of the individual becomes seriously altered in form, temperament and impulses. Since it is directly absorbed into the blood, these secretions are termed as internal secretions.

In the seminal discharge the male sperms formed in the testes are the vital elements because these sperms have the power of fertilising the egg of the woman to conceive a new life. These highly vitalized cells consist of a head, neck and long tail. It is in this head that the nucleus is contained which transmit the hereditary characteristics of the individual. Having the power of independent motion these sperms propel themselves in the liquid secretion in which it floats, it requires an hour or more for the sperm to reach the cavity of the uterus and a few hours to gain the oviduct or the tube where it fertilises an ovum (egg). When the released female egg encounters one male sperm or spermatozoa it penetrates the cell wall of the egg in a complex series of rearrangement of both cells, known as fertilisation. Though, in single male organism about 200 to 500 million sperms are discharged, only one is able to reach the walls of the cell. The remaining cells are cast out along with the other residues of the physiological process. The spermatozoa are being slowly formed and released in the testicles all the time.

Epididymis and Vas Deferens

Each of the cluster of convoluted tubes in the lobes of the testes in which the sperm cells are formed merges into a single tube and the resulting mass of tubes in turn forms a complex network which constitutes a large annexe to the body of the testes. It is known as epididymis. The network of the tubes of epididymis unite in turn to form the seminal duct or vas defrens. From the epididymis each seminal duct passes upwards in the scrotal sac and enters the pelvis cavity where it continues its upward course, then curves forward and downward to enter the urethra which conducts the urine from the bladder.

Seminal Vesicles

The vas two in number, issuing from each testes takes a round of the bladder and then empty into the seminal vesicles. These vesicles are two small pouches, situated just behind the urinary bladder. The function of seminal vesicles is to store the semen and secret a gelatinus substance which by mixing with the sperm thickens the semen and increases its volume. The secretion, the sperm thickens the semen and increases its volume. The secretion also provides nourishment and strength to sperms.

Since these testes and seminal vesicles are always secreting and manufacturing semen, sometimes the vesicles are filled to capacity and the nature empties them in the form of nocturnal emissions as is in the process orgasm. The phenomenon is usually accompanied by erotic dreams and pleasurable sex feelings of an orgasm.

It is a mistaken belief of old theories that nocturnal emissions or wet dreams are a sign of weaknes. These are natural, harmless occurrence to be expected in most normal men particularly between the ages of fourteen and thirty-five. There is nothing to worry about. Untold mental torture and unnecessary expense has been caused to millions of men through the misrepresentation of quacks and fear of men in these matters.

Seminal emissions vary greatly in frequency of occurrence between different men and in the same man at different times. Within the normal the frequency may range between once a month to several times a week . Many factors, physical, mental and temperamental–are responsible for it. There are some young men who rarely or never experience nocturnal emissions. Though the occurrence of emissions are natural, their absence does not necessarily indicate any abnormality. It is quite possible in their case that the contents naturally ooze out in the ducts aided by bowel movements, to be thrown out with the urine from the bladder.

Nocturnal emissions generally occur when a man sleeps on his back. The reason being that in this position the weight of the partly filled or full bladder resting upon the vesicles increases the irritation to set of the reflexes ejuculating semen. To avoid this, heavy food should not be taken before going to bed and constipation should not be allowed.

Prostate Gland

It is shaped like a horse chest nut. Surrounding the neck of the bladder and the junction of the urinary and spermatic ducts, into which juncture the prostate empties its contents through some thirty outlets. The prostrate secretion is also added to the semen before it is ejaculated in the vagina. Thus semen is a combined product of all these glands. Each of these glands imparts to the semen its many peculiar characteristics. The prostate is also a sexual gland, which is situated below the urinary bladder. During coital climax, the prostate cntracts and mixes its own secretion in the semen. To sustain sexual vigour and strength, it is considered necessary that the prostate functions properly. The prostate secretes a thin milky, alkaline fluid the function of which is similar to the products of the vesicles. The alkalinity serves to protect the spermatozoa against acidity arising from the urine. The acidity damages the vitality of the sperm cells.

Urethra

A small duct called urethra runs through the centre of the penis down to its glands from the urinary bladder. This duct serves the double purpose–it empties the urine from the bladder and ejaculates the semen from the seminal vesicles. Thus, urethra is connected with both the systems of seminal discharge and urine elimination. The urethra in penis discharges both semen and urine but sex mechanism of male body is such that both the actions cannot take place together. During seminal discharge a special valve automatically shuts off the urine.

Penis

A child's penis is small which grows long with the other organ of the body after the onset of puberty. Penis through which the bladder is emptied and the sperm is discharged during intercourse, is normally three to four inches long and in normal flaccid state about one and a quarter to two inches in diameter. When a man is sexually aroused his penis grows erect and organ measures about one and a half inches in diameter and five and half to six and a half inches in length along its upper side. It is made up in part of spongy tissue which becomes gorged with blood, making the organ hard and rigid . In excited state it stands out at an angle from the body to confirm in general to the normal vagina angle of the woman . The erection is essential in order to achieve the penetration of the vagina. In response to mechanical or psychic stimulation, the erction is achieved through a nervous mechanism which causes a rush of blood into the organ and at the same time greatly restricts its flow thus, causing rigid distention of the penis, Like the size, the shape also varies from man to man. Penis is the male copulating organ which conducts the semen into vagina. There is no correlation betwen the size of a penis and a man's sexual strength and capacity. The erect size also does not make much difference because vagina has such an elastic cavity to accommodate any size of penis. The most sensitive nerve ending in a vagina is the clitoris which can always be reached by any penis howsoever it be small.

Glans Penis

The foremost end of the penis round like a knob is called glans penis. It is slight thicker than the rest of the shaft. In the flaccid state of the penis the head or glans penis is partly or wholly by a loose layer of the skin, in the uncirumcised, called the prepuce of foreskin. This is retract for the purpose of cleaning and it becomes natural retracted after entry in coitus. The surface of the foreskin is somewhat mucus owing to the glans which secrete a substance called smegna. It is an irritating secretion and should be regularly cleaned, otherwise it makes the forepart of the penis become chessy in appearance by breeding germs. It should be daily washed with soap. The glans penis has the most sensitive nerve endings. A slight soft touch is enough to excite a man and to make the penis erect. It is mainly the glans penis on which a little rubbing whether by hand or by vaginal contact sends the sex waves in the entire body, culminating in orgasm or ejaculation.

Erection and Ejaculation

As also referred to earlier, the effect of the sexual arousal in man is physically manifest in the erection of the penis. A direct and gentle stimulation of the penis almost always causes erection. This is borne out of reflex action and may occur in sleep. Erection may be caused without any rubbing of the penis, just by erotic thoughts or dreams it goes erect. In the early morning it may be aroused because of the urge to urinate. Most such erections terminate without any discharge.

Ejaculation is the culmination of sexual stimulation in man. Having entered the vagina, the most sensitive nerve endings of which the penis is made up, become tense and excited on account of the friction against the walls of vagina, the cozy heat it may experience further fanned by the secretion of the fluid in the vagina. To and fro movements of the penis add on the arousal. The tension gets higher and higher till it reaches the climax and the release of the seminal fluids is known as ejaculation. The basic difference between the sex mechanism of the man and the woman is, in man the climax and ejaculation or orgasm take place simultaneously while in woman these are two different states. At the time of the climaxic height orgasm the seminal discharge takes place through the penis in a number of spurts.The number of the spurts varies from 4 to 20 just as the first menses indicates the onset of puberty in a girl,the first ejaculation marks the boy's entrance into adolescence.

Female Organs

The female organs are more complicated because they are confined in the body and not openly visible. Because of the apparent invisibility most of the girls are unaware about their internal sex organs. Hence , it is all the more necessary that full knowledge about the female organs structure and their function be discussed in full details.

Vulva

The two visibly fleshy folds, covered with hair are the outer lips or labia majora. When parted they reveal two smaller or inner lips of labia. The insides of the inner labia are covered with mucous membrnae. The inner lips or labia are one of the several sexual sensation centres. In sexual intercourse these labia remain constantly massaged by the rubbing of penis. In some women the inner lips protrude somewhat. The inner lips meet their upper ends which when separated look like the form of wish bone of a hen.

The principle of the sex feeling, the clitoris is situated just above the junction of the inner lips. The clitoris looks like a mini penis having erectile tissue and a head and foreskin similar to the penis of the man. It is covered from above by a hood of skin. The clitoris is made up of highly sensitive nerves which respond very well to sexual stimulation. It is from this centre that the sexual feeling begins and permeates in the entire body through vulva and vagina. When erect the clitoris looks like the size of or shape of small bean. About an inch below the clitoris is a small opening of the tube called urethra. Its duct conducts the urine from the bladder. The urethra has only the urinary function and no sexual function.

The muscous membrane above the clitoris , like the penis of a man, is covered with glands which secrete smegna. Owing to the structure, cleanliness in the woman is somewhat more difficult than it is in the man.

It is not hygeinically necessary to keep it clean but also for this reason that it emits smell which tend to inhbit sexual desire in the man.

Hymen

Just below the urinary passage is the entrance to vagina. In the normal virgin girl this opening remains partially close by a thin membrane called the hymen. Though it appears in different shapes but normally it looks like a crescent in shape appearing the forward extension of the black walls of the vagina. In many cases during the first intercourse when the hymen is ruptured there may be slight bleeding and pain. But this should not cause any alarm. It is a false notion which the orthodox still maintain that the hymen is the symbol of virginity. A nicked or stretched or tattered hymen does not mean that the body has been penetrated into. It could be ruptured on account of many a jerks or falls that a young girl might have experienced. Many girls may not have much of it or others may lose it in doing some kind of vigorous job. Sometimes the insertion of a finger into the vagina may prove too hard for any hymen. Occasionally a hymen is so tough that it remains intact even after several sessions of sexual intercourses. It all depends on the kind of hymen a girl is born with. Generally during the first coitus, the penis tear it till hardly a few shreds mark it former presence. At times in certain cases it was found to be so flexible that instead of breaking into pieces by the penile thrust, it merely bends and allows the penis to glide over it. It may in certain cases remain there even after delivering a child. In some cases the surgeon's aid is obtained to slit open the membrane. But the bleeding and discomfort, when they occur are not of sufficient consequence to warrant fear on the part of the woman. This is psychologically important because this fear powerfully inhibits her sexual responses and the function of the lubricating glands, leaving the parts dry. This increases the probability of discomfort and bleeding and diminishes the possibility of experiencing any sex pleasure at the first coitus.

Vagina

It is a tube or canal extending from vulva to the neck of the uterus. It is three and half to four inches in length in its normal relaxed position. It is here that the penis in intercourse is sheathed with its elastic walls. It receives the seminal discharge and allows the sperm to travel forward towards the womb in search of the ovum. It is through this tube that a child passes to the outside world during pregnancy. The vagina and its outlet becomes capable to great expansion, permitting the passage of the child from the womb without injury in many cases. In most instances, however more or less laceration of the muscular structure controlling the opening and of the vagina itself occurs. It should be vitally important that such tears receive prompt surgical attention. The use and control of the muslces about the vaginal opening of the entire pelvic floor are necessary to woman's most effective participation in coitus. The relaxed condition and the loss of muscular control which results from the failure to repair perineal and vaginal tears may result in greatly diminishing sexual satisfaction in coitus for both partners and may render it impossible for the woman to achieve orgasm at all. The flexible walls of the vagina are lined moist and clean. It has a great relaxing and contracting power. It is because of this reason that the vagina, besides being made up of flexible walls, is able to accommodate most larger penis not withstanding its small cavity.

Womb or Uterus

It is pear shaped organ of heavy muscular walls. The virgin uterus measures about two inches wide. Its elastic muscles expand considerably during pregnancy with the growth of the baby. Its upper part is connected with ovaries by two ducts called fallopian tubes. The organ is supported in the pelvis by strong ligaments, its position is at right angles to the vagina, the upper, heavy end being directed forward towards the front of the pelvis. The small end opens into the vagina and closes its upper end. After childbirth the organ gradually retracts to its normal size. The organ has powerful muscles to help push the baby out through the vagina. During pregnancy, the uterus retains and supplies nourishment to the growing baby till the delivery.

Fallopian Tubes and Ovaries

The upper end of the uterus as referred earlier are joined by the fallopian tubes, each about five and half inches long, which extend right and left to the ovaries. The function of the fallopian tube is to conduct ovum from the ovaries to the uterus. This is achieved through contractile action of the tubes finger like fringes called fimbria. The sweeping motion of fimbria is in one direction, which helps the egg cells in moving towards uterus. In most cases, the fertilisation of an egg cell or ovum takes place during its journey through the fallopian tube . The process of passing an egg cell through the tube is called ovulation. The fertilised egg is then moved down the tube towards the womb.

The ovaries can be compared likened to the testes of the male. They produce the female reproductive cells, the ova (eggs) and internal secretions. Situated at the outer ends of the tubes, one on each side of the uterus, an ovary is about the size and shape of a large almond in the shell. Though they are comparable to the testes in their function, the hormone function of the ovaries is apparently more complex than that of the testes of the male. In addition to the internal secretion which governs development of the specific female character and help to sustain the normal functioning of the individual as an organism, the ovaries elaborate other chemical substances which control the reproductive functions. If the ovaries are removed before puberty the development of the individual gets drastically altered. Even after marriage, if ovary is removed for any reason, there could be certain changes felt physically and mentally.

When a girl is born, her ovaries already contain these egg cells or ova in tens of thousands. But then these are not mature. With the onset of puberty the ovaries start their work of maturing ovum. During the life time of woman about 400 --500 of egg cells mature. From the time of puberty till menopause, every month a mature egg is produced by one of the ovaries. The mature egg cell passes through the fallopian tube towards the uterus. If an egg is fertilised it starts growing before it enters the velvety lined uterus which nourishes the egg well. If the egg is not fertilised it remains alive for about 20-44 hours after entering the tube and then it disintegrates and gets absorbed into the body. In that case soft and velvety lining of uterus is not required, the blood and the blood vessels forming the protective lining are cast out through vagina.

Menstruation

When the egg cell is not fertilised, the monthly preparation by the womb to receive a fertilised egg cell gone a waste and the debris is cast out–the whole process is known as menstruation. Menstruation generally continues for three to five days but even longer in few cases. While it is a normal physiological function, not to be regarded as a 'sickness' or being 'unwell'. In several cases the general let down and the readjustments of the entire organism do involve nervous tensions and in many cases a variety of aches and pains for which due allowance is to be made in the social and personal circle of the individual. It should be clearly understood that a girl or woman during the periods, should not be considered an 'untouchable' . As a matter of fact, the underlying reason of this belief was sympathetic–that in a period of menstruation, a girl or a lady might feel weak so she should be given full rest–which has been mistakenly converted into a hygienic one. But now a days no educated girl or woman adhere to these obscurantic norms and treat the period days like any other day in their life. May be, because of better facilities to contain this blood into the sanitary napkins, the modern woman does not make a show of it. It is not physically but emotionally a woman might feel disturbed during this period, for which she should be shown due consideration.

Breasts

Though the breasts do not strictly come under the categories of the organs we are discussing, they are being induced because of their special significance in manifestation of the sexual arousal of a woman. Specially their breasts' nipples signify as one of the most erogenous zones on woman's body. Squeezing, sucking, touching, caressing of the breasts, particularly the nipples give rise to strong and most favourable sexual desires. The sexologists say that in the initial stages of married life a woman derives more pleasure from any such stimulation of her breast than the actual coitus. Nipples, like clitoris have erectile tissues and very sensitive nerve endings. The tissues become firm and erect during erotic stimulation. It is for this reason that breasts or mammary glands are two very important sexual organs, whose development is dependent on the secretion of certain hormones of the female sex. Though, the breasts have their primary function in feeding a new born child, there importance as an erotic and sensitive zone permeating with desire to mate has great significance in sexual relationship. Although their sizes vary from puberty to maturity and they grow large during pregnancy. The sexual undertones of this organ has influenced the loving onlookers most. An ideally formed breast has always been the most beautiful female symbol or characteristic. The another most important function of breasts is to feed child after delivery.

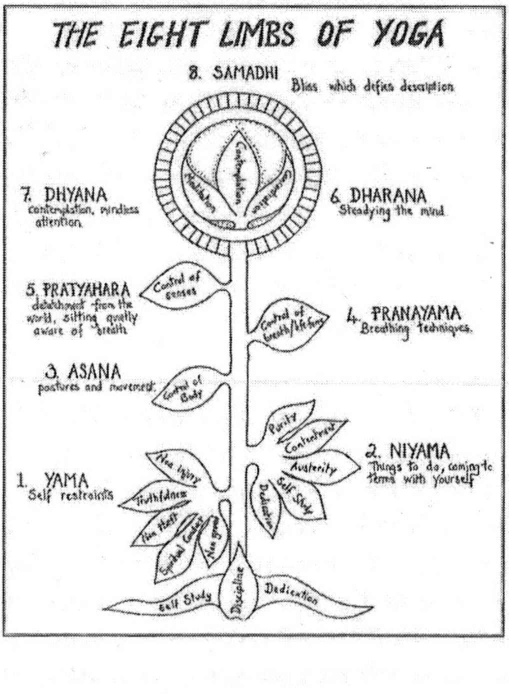

□□□□

2.
SOME IMPORTANT POINTS BEFORE STARTING YOGIC EXERCISES

Of all the complementary or alternate therapies yoga is the most cost effective, holistic, curative, hassle-free and easy-to-perform. It not only purifies body, mind and intellect but, apart from that, it strives to improve digestive, respiratory, cardiac and circulatory, endocrine glands' functioning, mobility and sleeplessness of joints and muscles, renders body slim and trim by helping it to shed extra fat from the body, activates sebaceous glands to keep the skin glazed and sparkling, improves health of ovaries, controls senses. I have mentioned only some of the benefits.

Yogasanas are not aerobic or physical exercises, or work-up for sportsmen and athletes, but much more than that. There is hardly any mental and physical disorder (*Dosha* or *Roga*) which it cannot cure, of course it has to be coupled with Pranayama Kriyas to derive optimum and near complete mileage. Readers are advised to go through the following points carefully so that no room is left for confusion.

Yoga and Food

Yoga lays great stress on pure non-irritant, spice free, anti-toxicant, and fresh seasonal vegetable and fruits. Hence, pure vegetarian diet is an integral part of this unique system. Try to avoid fried, saucy, spicy, fat-enriched diet which interferes not only with normal functioning of body organs but also disturbs our mental faculties, thinking, secretions from endocrine glands –in a way all these factors are health hazards. It has been rightly said that 'we are what we eat' which clearly implies that our food patterns and dietary habits not only govern our body but also our thinking process. When our body is ailing, mind is bound to get disturbed, as healthy mind stays only in a healthy body and, in order to keep our body in a healthy state, our diet must be 'Sattvik'. For instance, if a person consumes much of spicy and fat-enriched food, alcohol, tobacco, drugs, his digestive system is bound to get disturbed, resulting in many digestion related disorders.

Yoga and Mind

Mind is the driving force of all our actions. If mind is vitiated, polluted and disturbed, our endocrine glands won't function normally–there will be lessor or more secretion from such glands which will adversely affect our body chemistry. Yoga strives to pacify agitated mental process, thereby imparting it peace, tranquillity and satiation. Yogic postures assist the brain to put in better performance, by nurturing its nerves with the requisite blood supply to sustain and fortify its various activities. Mind is an abstract form of brain and whatever thoughts arise therein are expressed by emotions, sensations, physical actions or reactions.

Yoga and Pranayama

Pranayama means suspension or withholding of breath or regulation of breath through inhalation. Suspension (withholding) and exhalation, and these three phases are part and parcel of all the yogic postures (asanas). There is life as long as we breathe and death ensues only when last breath comes out of our body. If one is able to retain breath, the time saved through retention, adds to longevity of life. Prana is nothing other than breath, hence in order to add to years, one must learn how to preserve expense of breath.

Yogasanas are designed in such a way that entire body's functions get normalised, breathing process regulated, quality of life improved and general well-being of body, mind and intellect ensured. A person who practises yogasanas and pranayama with punctual regularity can be rest assured to lead a healthy, physical and mental life.

All asanas cannot and must not be performed by all, due to variable disorders and an individual's physical capacity, but Pranayama can be practised by all persons, irrespective of age, sex and physical condition.

Multiple Benefits of Yogasans

Asanas have multiple benefits, as detailed hereunder –

1. With certain safeguards and cautions, all men, women and children can perform asanas, depending upon an individual's age, health status or particular diseases from which a person is suffering.
2. They are easy, cost-effective, preventive, corrective and curative of almost all the disorders, mental or physical or both, and no extra material is required to perform them.
3. They help in muscle and tissue build-up and repair thereof, apart from calming down agitated nerves, dispelling fatigue, making up for the lost energy. They help to keep body and mind in good humours.
4. They energise the endocrine glands so that the body receives requisite sections which are vital and necessary for proper functioning of the body.
5. Digestive system is rejuvenated, appetite improved, digestion related diseases are cured.
6. It is the best method to keep and sustain flexibility of the spine and remove curvature, if any. In addition, it also rectifies posture-related diseases like back pain, shoulder pain, cervical spondylosis, lumbar spondylosis, joint pains, stiffness of joints etc.

7. Asanas help to reduce weight, by naturally shedding extra flesh from the body.

8. They sharpen intellect, enhance memory and agility, provide suppleness and strength to mind, enabling it to concentrate / meditate. All the mental faculties and systems get renewed energy, vigour. Higher values of mind are also aroused.

9. They tone up the body, from top to bottom, regulate respiration, control cardiac, pulmonary, urinary and digestive systems in such a perfect way that hardly any room is left for malfunctioning. They also purify and regulate circulation of blood, by fortifying lungs and heart.

10. Each and every organ of the body is recharged and activated. Nervous system is toned up and diseases like hypertension, cardiac complications, mental tensions, stress, anger, agitation, approach to life are dispelled. In a way, where other therapies miserly fail and raise their hand up in despair, yoga solves them in the shortest time and, above all, the sufferer feels relieved without any trace of side-effects.

11. Those who practise the asanas regularly, improve their eyesight and, in certain cases, one may give up the use of aspects even or else his number may, at least, fall.

12. Skin becomes soft , glossy, tender and strong enough to withstand thermic changes. Sudden weather changes have no or very little impact on the practice of Asanas.

13. Facial wrinkles vanish, complexion improves, signs of old age disappear and one feels to have gained a renewed vigour, vitality and glow. Rigid joints attain flexibility and mobility, especially flexibility of spine, which is necessary to retain and sustain youth. An old man even attains innocence and agility of a child.

14. Asanas provide immunity against diseases, and also arouse prophylaxis.
15. Other systems merely aim at toning up the body whereas yogasanas provide multifold benefits due to the fact that there are specific asanas for each and every disorder, whether physical or mental.

Importance of Yogic exercises as compared to other games or exercises

- Yogic exercises are very good for the exercise of internal organs of the body; like liver, pancreas, intestines, lungs, heart, kidneys, spine and joints etc. In other exercises the internal organs are not exercised upto that level, as in Yogic exercises.
- In yoga the muscles are relaxed, heart beats are in perfect rhythm and the mind calm and peaceful as there is no competition while performing yoga, where as in sports, there is anxiety and stress due to competition.
- Yoga can be discontinued due to illness or certain other reasons with no side effects or weight gain, whereas if games or other exercises are discontinued, there are chances of weight gain and lethargy.

Know About Precautions

- These exercises should not be performed by severely ill persons or who are bed ridden or suffering from acute slip disc pain or having a fracture.
- Females during pregnancy and menstruation should avoid and if required, perform only under supervision of an experienced yoga teacher.
- Children below the age of five years should not perform Yogic exercises, as their internal organs are very tender.
- If you are suffering from chronic ailments like arthritis, migraine, diabetes, renal failure, slip disc, cirrhosis of liver

etc., perform these exercises only under supervision of a good yoga teacher.

- If you feel any pain during a particular exercise, stop doing that.
- If you feel exhausted, do 'Shavasana' at once, as this asana can be performed after any asana. Otherwise this particular asana is advised to be performed in last.

❑❑❑❑

3.
FACTORS NECESSARY FOR PERFORMANCE OF YOGASANAS

Yoga is not exclusively meant for the benefits of saints, asctics and mystics. It, in fact, serves to benefit all and one alike but the benefits and time taken to attain the desired result will depend on sincerity, regularity, patience and will to learn and perform. Burning desire to learn is the main driving force behind yoga, besides faith and confidence.

It is a complete, dependable and time-tested discipline and to derive optimum benefits, following points deserve to be borne in mind.

One should not nurture any ill-will, tension or inimical feeling. Apply yourself fully in the yogic sadhana and practice, forgetting worries and cares. Your mind should be in a happy and peaceful state, while you embark upon performing asanas. Try to overcome what ails you, physically and mentally.

Time

Ideal time to perform asanas is the early morning time, preferably before sunrise. Attend to the calls of nature and do not take anything before and after the exercises. If, however, morning time does not suit, asanas can be performed in the evening time also but nothing should be taken 3-4 hours prior to performing yogic kriyas. While doing yoga do not exert undue strain on your limbs. Initially, due to lack of practice and rigidity of joints and muscles, it may take a bit longer time but, as the time passes, all such problems would disappear or, at best, show a declining trend for the better. Have patience; do not be cruel to your body as it will require some time to adjust itself to respond and withstand the demands made on it. It is not wise to change timings so be punctual and regular.

Place

Neat, clean, open, fresh environs are the prerequisites for yogic practice. Polluted, contaminated and unnatural environs will do more harm. If latter is the case, it is better to bid good-bye to such a practice, till such time as you are able to find suitable site. Open, green and clean gardens or countryside or bank or river are perhaps the most ideal places which are amiss in modern big cities. Instead, you can utilise your terrace for the purpose or else well ventilated rooms, where fresh air can enter without any disturbance. Proper place, light, open and fresh air, a soft blanket mat should always be handy. In winter you may use even a mattress or else a quilt may be used.

After completing an asana, give rest to your nerves, rather to whole body, and performing of shavasana (corpse posture / pose) would meet this requirement. Rest is necessary for the tired body and before you switch on to another asana, there should be a reasonable gap.

Rest

Whenever after doing an asana, you ever feel tired, at once suspend the asana and give proper rest to your body. Whenever, during course of an asana, you feel your body is getting tired and that you are unable to carry forward or continue any asana anymore, at once start relaxing your body. Fatigue is a warning signal from nature, warning you that as the optimum exertion has already of any consequence, what matters is how much mileage you have derived in the minimum of time span.

Bath

Bathing is not merely a ritual, it is also intended to purify the body. Bathing opens pores of the body also, when it is vigorously rubbed with a towel. If bath is taken before yoga postures, it would render the body light and also help on facilitating the process of asana. You can take bath with hot water, even after the asana is over, but a gap of 30 minutes is all the more necessary. Make sure that you towel your body in such a way that there is no moisture left on your body.

Dress

The dress used for the asanas should conform to weather conditions but, it must be ensured, that body is not overloaded with too much of clothes, as it will create problems while you are performing the asanas. Try to wear minimum of the clothes, but not so spared as to expose your body to ravages of atmosphere. Always wear loose clothes, as tight ones would restrict free movement of limbs. Ladies may use salwar-kameez or slacks and men underwears, trousers or half pants for the performance of asanas.

Breakfast

There should ideally be a gap of half-an-hour between asanas and breakfast. Take only light and easily digestible breakfast and should not be so much to fill your belly to the full. Avoid taking any cold drink or food immediately after an asana is over. If you wish, you may have a glassful of milk (Hot).

Sun-Bath

It will always be handy. In winter you may use even a mattress or else a quilt may be used.

After completing an asana, give rest to your nerves, rather to whole body, and performing of shavasana (corpse posture) would meet this requirement. Rest is necessary for the tired body and, before you switch on to another asana, there should be a reasonable gap.

General

All the asanas are based on and named after parts of the body, material objects, and animals. There are innumerable asanas but, in practice only 84 asanas are said to meet all the disorders which afflict all persons, in one way, or at one time or the other. Asanas are not medicines or tonics, they tend to correct the wrongs done by us. They also awaken our auto-immune mechanism which is adversely affected by various factors. They correct the defective metabolism, inducing and fortifying the fighting capacity of our body to drive out the invading forces. They aim at rooting out the cause of the malady which often emanates from disturbance of the mind.

4.
ASANAS AND DISEASES (DISORDERS)

Asanas and Diseases (Disorders)

Hereunder, we are giving a list of asanas which are useful to cure a particular disease. The practitioner can perform and choose from them, according to his need, capacity and convenience. Asanas for most common diseases only are being mentioned against individual diseases.

1. Cold: Sarvangasana, Halasana, Shirshasana.
2. Cough: Matsyasana, Janushirasana, Supat vajrasana, Urdhavajrasana.
3. Asthma: Shirshasana, Shavaasana, Sarvaangasana, Matsyasana, Supatvajrasana, Shalabhasana, Ushtrasana and Ujjayi Pranayma.
4. Diabetes: Dhanurasana, Matsyendrasana, Naukasana, Surya Namaskarasana, Sarapasana (Cobra Bhujangasana).
5. Stomach Disorders: Sukhasana, Padmasana, Bhujangasana, Ardhachakraasana, Uttaanpadaasana, Shalabhasana.
6. Liver Disorders: Mayurasana, Bhujangasana, Shalbhasana, Shirshasana, Shashankasana, Halasana, Ushtrasana.
7. Mental Tension: Trikonasana, Halasana Vajrasana, Shavasana, Garbhasana, and Sarvangasanas.

8. Nervous Debility: Hala, Chakra, Dhanur, Garbha, Vajra, Sarvaang, Shalabh, Pashchimttaanasana, Sheetal and Sheetkari Pranayama.
9. Nervous Tension: Shava and Koormasanas.
10. Insomnia : Hala and Shirshaasana, Sarvaangasana, Sheetal and Sheetkari Pranayama.
11. Hypertension (Acute): Shashaank, Vajra and Pawan Muktasanas.
12. Kidney problems: Ardha matsyendra, Ushtra, Bhujang, Gomukh, Shashaank, Hala and Dhanurasanas.
13. Obesity: Trikone, Paschimuttaan, Dhanur, Hala, Shalabh, Sarvaang, Paad Hastaasana, Nari Shodhan, Udyan Bandh Asana.
14. Pain in joints (Arthritis): Trikone, Santula, Gomukh, Sidha, Natraj, Veer, Vrikhsha and Setubandha Asanas.
15. Back Pain: Chakra, Dhanur, Bhujang, Mayur, Shashanka, Vajrasuputra, Padma, Trikone, Utkat, Nauka and Padshalab asana.
16. Rheumatism: Dhanur, Padam and Vajra Asanas.
17. Spinal Disorders: Hala, Dhanur, Chakra, Bhujang, Sheersha, Vrischik, Shashank, Ushtra, Pashchimuttaan asanas.
18. Gout: Dhanur, Paschimuttaan, Pawanmukta, Trikone, Parvat, Gomukh, Ardhamatsyendra, Janushir asanas.
19. Sciatica: Vajra, Gomukh and Hanuman asanas.
20. Constipation: Tadha, Chakra, Janushira, Mayur, Bhujang, Dhanur, Bhoomi-Pada-Mastak, Supta-Vajra, Karna-Peerhan, Pada hasta, Matsya asanas.
21. Worms: Nauka, Vrishchik, Matsyendra, Mayur, Sarvang, Shirsha, Paschimottaan, asanas.

22. Acidity: Shalabh asana.
23. Sour Eructations: Bhujang, Janushir, Chakra, Ushtra, Hasta-Pada-nghustha, Pashchimuttaan asanas.
24. Frigidity and Sterility : Bhujang, Shirsha, Paschimattaan, Sarvang, Matsaya and Supatvajrasanas.
25. Weak Sexual Power: Chakra, Sarvanga, Garurn, Vatayan, Bhujang, Pashchimottaan, Shirsha asanas.
26. Coryza : Shirsha, Hala and Sarvanga asanas.
27. Throat Infections: Singha, Sarvang, Shirsha, Hala, Chakra, Bhujang, Suptavajra and Matsayaasanas.
28. Menstrual Disorders: Hala, Dhanur, Shava, Vajra, Sarvanga, Bhujang, Matsya, Parvat, Shalabh and Shirshasanas.
29. Piles and Fistula: Sidha, Gomukh, Bhadra, Chandra, Namaskar, Janushira, Sukh, Saravnga, Uttanpada asanas.
30. Fatigue: Shava, Matsya and Dand asanas.

Note - There is hardly any mental and / or physical disorder which yoga cannot cure and above list only refers to common disorders only, other disorders are too many to be detailed here, for want of space.

As for practice of asanas is concerned, it is advised that some authentic book is studied, and its contents fully read and learnt. To begin with, the prospective adherent must seek guidance from a yoga expert who would clearly explain the 'Do' s and Don't's' of relevant and requisite asanas, with special reference to a particular disease for the eradication and cure of which a particular yogic asana is desired / recommended to be practised. The asanas, which we have referred to, in relation to particular disorders, are called 'Swasthya Asanas' which are secondary to 'Dhayana Asana' which enjoy superior status because the latter ones aim at controlling wavered tendencies of mind, aids in controlling the mind, helps in meditation and concentration.

For the efficient and proper performance of all the asanas, which are meant for the proper maintenance of body in a healthy state, only a yoga teacher can guide. But, for the benefit of readers, we are giving hereunder very prominent asanas which, hopefully, would strive to serve the mankind.

□□□□

5.
ROOT CAUSE OF ALL PROBLEMS – ENERGY IMBALANCE

Disease of any kind whether physical, mental or psychosomatic indicates some imbalance inside us. This imbalance is nothing but imbalance in the energy body. It is interesting to note that this life energy or prana is linked both to body and mind. It is an intermediary or bridge between the two and this only explains how physical body affects the non physical mind and how non physical mind affects the body.

Anything happening in the body also affects the mind through the agency of prana. Similary, anything happening in the mind also affects the body through the agency of prana. Hence body and mind are functioning in a healthy manner, energy or prana is flowing freely and uniformly everywhere. There is no blockage, congestion or depletion of prana anywhere. Hence there is no disease.

However, when body and mind are being misused, functioning unhealthy, abnormally or are overexerted, energy flow becomes imbalanced, i.e. energy becomes blocked and congested at one place, depleted at another place leading to some kind of disease (dis-ease) in body.

Physical Factors Causing Imbalance

Now at the bodily level there are many factors by which we disturb the natural and healthy functioning of energy body.

Some of them are listed below:

1. Irregular lifestyle (e.g. sleeping, walking, eating at irregular and odd timings).
2. Overeating, oversleeping.
3. Use of alcohol, smoking (tobacco), tea, coffee, narcotic drugs.
4. Faulty diet (Rajasik and Tamsik foods).
5. Overexertion.
6. Overindulgence in sensual pleasures.
7. Excessive talking/gossiping/roaming unnecessarily.
8. Faulty postures, faulty breathing.
9. Living in polluted, noisy environment. Living in extremely hot/cold/humid environment.
10. Excessive company and mingling with people.
11. Drugs and medication.

In short, if any Rajasik or Tamsik activity disturbs the energy flow of the body then it generates negative energy. On the other hand, Satwik lifestyle and activities promote the balanced and free flow of prana and generate positive energy. Whatever organs or systems get damaged due to the negative physical factors mentioned above, pranic flow in the corresponding nadis and chakras get disturbed.

Mental Factors Causing Imbalance

As mentioned earlier, just like physical factors, mental factors can also affect energy flow and damage chakras. If we want to sum up all the negative mental factors in two words, which disturb the flow of prana and health of chakras, those two words will be 'Negative thinking'. Now the next question comes 'why negative thinking arises'? The simple answer is –not accepting and understanding the things as they really are. The more the gap between the reality of things and your imagination/assumption about them, the more tense, nervous and anxious you will be.

Because of this huge gap between how things really are and what we imagine them to be, we are continually suppressing, rejecting and fighting with ourselves and outside world. This doesn't allow us to be integrated, whole and complete in our personality. We become a fragmented personality where one protion is going this way, another portion is going that way and third portion is another way. The result is tension and conflict which does't allow energy to flow freely. As per yoga psychology, in such a state our unconsciousness is relatively vast and consciousness not well developed.

So, the first thing to do is to stop suppressing things and start seeing and understanding things from a broader perspective. We should start accepting and integrating everything into our consciousness avoiding nothing. This integration finally leads us to a state of unity, wholeness and completeness. Suppression brings about separation which creates loneliness, discomfort and a feeling of dis-ease. Whatever is suppressed and not integrated into our personality becomes alien to us and a constant source of disturbance. But as we develop, a process of integration takes place among all alienated or conflicting aspects of ourselves leading to increased happiness and satisfaction.

When our consciousness is fully developed, we finally reach that state of enlightenment and equilbrium from which all can be understood, appreciated and accepted. It is also to be noted that when consciousness is not fully developed and integrated, there is lot of egocentric move and selfishness in one's personality and lack of concern for others. But as consciousness gradually becomes expanded and integrated, we become less self-centred with more concern for others. This, in spiritual parlance, is also stated as moving from a state of separation (selfishness) to the state of unity (selflessness).

Now when the personality is not integrated, it is reflected in our behaviour in various forms as mentioned below:

(a) Negative emotions (e.g. anger, irritation, impatience, intolerance, fear, anxiety, worry, nervousness, hatred, jealousy, revengeful nature, hurry, over-ambition, restlessness, depression, sadness, hopelessness and helplessness, lack of confidence, etc.)

(b) Desires and expectations.

(c) Craving and passion for name, fame, power, status, control, domination.

(d) Various 'Vikaras' like greed, attachment, selfishness, ego, etc.

(e) Unsteadiness and distractions in mind, inability to focus.

Now the most important question is how these negative mental factors affect our energy body and then the physical body.

The explanation of this question is that these negative mental factors create corresponding vibrations in our astral body. Since astral body is connected to etheric body (or pranic body) at the point of chakras or energy centress, hence corresponding chakras get affected and start malfunctioning. Now the organs to which these chakras feed energy, also start malfunctioning as a result.

The following table shows the relationsip between the energy centress (or body part having this energy centre) and corresponding mental factors which influence them.

Mental Feeling

Energy centre which is affected

1. Inability to love all universally	Heart chakra will be blocked
2. Lack of self-expression, inability to communicate and speak effectively	Throat chakra will be blocked
3. Excessive sex and sensory pleasures	Hara chakra will be blocked

4.	Craving for name, fame, ego, power; domination and control over others; aggressiveness, anger, jealousy, hatred impatience; violence, cruelty, harshness exploitation	Solar plexus chakra will be blocked
5.	Compassion, love, kindness, sympathy	Heart chakra will be opened
6.	Fear, insecurity, feeling threat to survival for all, unity with creation knees, calves and feet will be affected (Refer Reiki positions)	Root chakra will be blocked
7.	Deep-rooted feeling of hurt and guilt	Hara and throat chakras will be affected
8	Foul speech, shouting, showing disrespect to others	Throat chakra will be blocked
9.	Humbleness and sweetness in talking with love and respect	Throat chakra will be opened
10.	Unsteadiness of mind and eyes	Ajna chakra will be blocked
11.	Inability to forgive enemies	Ajna chakra will be blocked
12.	Extreme helplessness and hopelessness	Paralysis, numbness of arms, hands and leg, Asthma
13.	Oversensitiveness, (Eczema, suppression restricted Acne etc.) communication between you and world	Allergy, skin problems

14. Steadiness/concentration of mind and eyes	Ajna chakra will be opened
15. Forgiveness	Ajna chakra will be opened
16. Greediness, attachment leading to constipation	Hara chakra will be affected
17. Disharmony and non adjustment in reationships with partner and close relatives resulting in disappointment, frustration	Kidneys will be affected
18. Pent-up aggression, bitterness, hard feelings	Gallstones, kidney stone will be formed.
19. Overthinking and overplanning	Swadhisthan (or Hara) chakra will be damaged
20. Feariessness	Mooladhara chakara will be opened.

Energy Imbalance From Yogic Perspective

In yoga, the energy balance is explained in terms of activity of Ida, Pingala and Sushumna nadis, and it is very interesting to know about it.

Imbalance towards Left Side

As has been explained earlier, Ida nadi (or moon's channel) travels along the left side of the spine starting from the Muladhara chakra and ascending upto Ajna chakra. The qualities assigned to this nadi are Tamoguna, past events and subconscious. It always brings to consciousness the memories of the past. The persons who are left sided (i.e. in whom Ida nadi mostly remains active) are those people who keep on thinking of the past, are very emotional, prefer darkness, avoid meeting people and are introverts. Such persons get various types of diseases of the left side. They become very lethargic, retreating into passivity and self obsession which finally culminates in lunacy, epilepsy, senile decay.

Persons who are left sided should balance it with the right side by activity, work and action, discarding all ideas of self destruction and self pity. Our left side is represented on the whole left hand.

Imbalance towards Right side

As has been mentioned, Pingala nadi or the sun channel runs along the right side of spine starting from Muladhara up to Ajna chakra. This nadi has qualities of Rajo Guna. It represents our desire for action (Kriya Shakti). It makes us think, work, plan and organize for the future events.

The symptoms of right sided persons are that they are very aggressive, over ambitious and dominating type. Right sided persons become very dry and lose all soft feelings. They are concerned only for their selfish material achievement and power over others. Blinded by ego, they take pride in exploiting and fooling the world. Such people get diseases of right side, problems on Pingala nadi result largely from our presumption that it is we who are doing something while in fact all work is done only by Almighty God.

Any extreme physical or mental activity can paralyze our left emotional side and move us on to the right side so that we move into supraconscious (future) where we see visions like those induced by hallucinogenic drugs.

Overactive right side is brought into balance by moving the energy towards the centre, to Satoguna, our right side is represented on our whole right hand.

Balance at the Centre

When the powers of both left (Ida nadi) and right side (Rajoguna) are brought to balance, we get established in the centre or Satoguna.

The central channel or Sushumna nadi begins at Mooladhara and goes straight up to the highest chakra namely 'Sahasrara'. The qualities of this nadi are Sato guna, present centredness and superconsciousness. It is represented in both the hands. It is through this channel that we become superconscious and integratd into one whole. When Sushumna nadi gets opened, Kundalini can ascend in this central channel and go right up to Sahasrara chakra leading to our enlightenment. Doing regular meditation in thoughtless awareness (pure perception) and leading virtuous life is vital to opening of Sushumna.

Sushumna nadi is also called the channel of the Eternal present, where the only time is not. In this way, we transcend time and space by opening of Sushumna and Kundalini awakening.

Achieving the Balance of Nadis

In 'Sahaj Yoga' some simple techniques are suggested to achieve the balancing of right and left sides of the body as mentioned below;

(i) If a person is right sided then the energy of Ida nadi is raised by making ascending movements of the right hand along the right side and brought to the left side or the person's spine .

(ii) If a person is left sided, i.e. apathetic and depressed, then the energy of Pingala nadi is raised by making ascending movements of the right hand along left side of the body and brought to the right side of the person's spine.

Clearing the Chakras

A chakra could also be cleared by simulating its clockwise rotation with the fingers of the right hand by a healer and asking the patient to keep his right hand on the afflicted chakra and keeping his left hand on the left knee with palms up and fingers open. In the science of prana, left hand is always used for receiving energy and right hand for imparting energy. Now depeding on which side of chakra is afflicted–whether left side, right side, front or back, there can be slight variations accordingly in the healing.

There are other methods of clearing the chakras also, e.g. candling. It clears the chakras on the left side. Here a burning candle is moved up and down on the left side of spine. Similarly, there are other methods for clearing chakras like foot soaking in lukewarm salt water. Right side chakras are normally cleared by cold water treatment in the form of foot soaking in cold water. Foot soaking in river or sea water is said to clear Solar and Hara chakras. Sitting on mother earth or walking barefoot on the earth or grass clears Muladhara chakra. Putting hands on earth or in flowing river water or in lukewarm salt water is equally beneficial for clearing chakras. Salt has the special quality of breaking down the negative energy. Doing concentration or "Trataka" with open eyes on some object especially candle flame helps in awakening the Ajna chakra. Even when in a normal way our mind is focussed and centered in some activity, it helps in activating Ajna chakra. Meditation is the strongest method for energizing Ajna chakra.

Yoga science also speaks of reciting (mentally) specific mantras for awakening each chakra. This science is based on matching the subtle frquency of each chakra with subtle frequency of specific mantra so as to create resonance. However, since the subject is Reiki, we won't go into these details in this book.

Another teachnique of clearing chakra is by strengthening their qualities as mentioned in the table of chakras. As has been mentioned earlier, the chakras which are catching and blocked are only responsible for psychic and physical problems.

One of the easiest method to awaken chakras is to mentally focus your attention (with eyes closed) on them. To increase your concentration on a particular chakra you can imagine that you are breathing through that chakra (i.e. inhaling and exhaling through that point).

All the above information for clearing nadis and chakras is given here only for general enlightenment of the reader. However, since the purpose of this book is to cleanse the energy body through Reiki healing , the other chapters have the details of healing your energy body through Reiki. Nevertheless if you continue to use other techniques for balancing your energy body as described in this chapter and also in chapter titled 'Supporting aids for Reiki Practive, it will definitely do you more good.

□□□□

6.
IMPORTANT YOGASANAS FOR EVERY ONE

Here is a description of yogasanas,which can be performed by anyone, but if you do these under guidance of some expert, it will be more beneficial.

Padmasana (Lotus Pose)

Method - It is called Padmasana because while performing it, legs appear in the form of a lotus. Sit on the ground and stretch forward your legs, keeping them together. Now left foot should be placed over the right thigh, and right foot over the left thigh, making sure that the heels touch the abdomen on both sides on the either side of nail. Keep the hands on the knees. Keep the head and back portion erect. Both the feet should touch the ground, and eyes be kept closed. This asana can be utilised for doing Pranayama. If you wish, you can join index finger and thumbs, base of thumb resting on index finger's nail, a sign of Mudra Pranayama.

Benefits - It is very useful to gain concentration of mind, to enhance mental faculties, to do mental work, especially useful for the aged person. It prevents trapping of wind in the body; preserves vital fluids of the body, imparts solace, peace, solitude and longevity. It tones up reproductive organs and system of females, prevents and cures abdominal disorders. For dhyana (meditation), padmasana is unique and ideal asana.

Vajrasana (Thunder bolt Posture)

Method - It is named thunderbolt, as it imparts the strength to body as if it is made like a stone or as strong as a thunder bolt. It is the only asana, in yoga, which can be practised after 45 minutes or more from the time of finishing your meals. In between meal times, it can also be done, but never immediately after meals. Kneel down on the floor, letting your big toes, and legs and knees touch the ground. Now rest your buttocks on your knees, your heels bent inwards and thumbs touching each other. Place the palms on the knees, keeping your spine erect but relaxed and flexible. Breathing should be even, deep and slow. Expand your chest, drawing the abdominal muscles inwards.

Benefits - This asana will expel gas and remove acidity. How much you have overeating, it will digest the same. It tones up sexual system of both males and females, removes pain and stiffness in spine and knees, lowers raised blood pressure, gives longevity and retards and postpones old age. For meditation, it is an ideal asana, as you can sit in this asana as long as you wish. After completion of this asana, simply massage with your hands or, still better, use salt mixed oil, say of mustard, which can be slightly luke-warmed.

Bhujang or Sarpasana (Cobra / Serpent Pose)

Method - Lie flat on the ground, abdominal portion touching the ground. Straighten both the arms, palms touching the ground. Now bring the palms at level with both sides of abdomen. Slowly lift your neck and torso in such a way that whole body rests on your palms. Now lift your neck upwards gradually and try to look upwards as far and as conveniently you can. Let the toes touch the ground and palms securely resting on the ground. Do not let your elbows bend down. Stay in the position as long you can. When you feel suffocated or when there is a feeling that you can't endure/continue any more, then slowly get back to original position from where you had started. After the asana is over, loosen your limbs and relax.

Benefits - Abdominal muscles and back portion are supplied with blood and blood circulation in general, is improved and also fresh and pure blood is supplied to all the organs. It imparts strength, flexibility and tone to spinal column. It removes menstrual disorders and irregularity, helps to improve digestion, chance of night discharge is dispelled, helps to maintain celibacy. It is useful for diabetics, as it activates the pancreas, thereby causing secretion of insulin, render arms, hands and neck painless, flexible and active. Kidneys and intestines also are strengthened. It removes obesity and sheds extra flesh from the abdominal portion, and spinal curvature and postural abnormalities are also removed.

Dhanurasana (Bow-Shaped Posture)

Method - Lie flat on the ground, your abdominal side touching the ground. Fold your legs from the knees. Now lift your neck and torso, gradually keeping your hands along sides of your back. Try to catch hold of your ankles with your hands. Gradually stretch your hands and feet so that they form a bow-shape, stay in this position as long as you can. Then regain the former position and relax by loosening your limbs.

Benefits - It has all the benefits detailed under Bhujangasana, as it is simply and extended form of the former. When you are doing Dhanurasana, there is hardly any need for practising Bhujangasana. Its added benefits are in strengthening of hands, elbows, ankles, knees. In short, both the lower and upper extremities become more flexible and strong, abdominal pressure helps in secretion of digestive juice and activities endocrine glands. In both these asanas, no jerk should be exerted on any organ. This suggestion is good for all other asanas too. Pregnant ladies must not perform this asana.

Gomukhasana (The Cow-Face Posture)

Method - Sit on the floor, keeping the legs stretched forward. Fold the left leg at the knee and sit on the left foot with the help of hands, fold the right leg and place the right thigh on the left thigh. Bring heels of both the feet together so that they touch each other which can be done by lifting your buttocks a bit. Now bend your right arm from the ear (right side) and bring the hand on the back side of your end. Fold the left hand behind your back and try to form a hook in which both the hands are clasped. Care should be taken not to over exert your limbs. Gradually you will get to the desired position as your limbs attain flexibility. Keep yourself in this position for about 30 seconds. Thereafter, give yourself some pause and reverse the position of hands and legs. If a lady wishes to develop her breast on a particular side, she should perform this asana more with the hand of that side (on which she wishes to develop her breast).

Benefits - This asana is equally beneficial for both the males and females, as it strengthens the muscle of shoulder, chest/ breast and makes legs stronger. Muscles of relevant organs are also rendered elastic. After completing the asana, whether on either or both sides, never strain your limbs. Initially, you may find it convenient to perform the asana on one side only, but regular practice will remove all the hesitancy and stiffness, thus making way for you to do the asana on the other side too.

Sarvangasana (Pan Physical Pose)

Method - Lie flat on the ground, your spine touching the floor, stretch the body, raise the legs slowly and let them stay at right angle to the trunk. After staying for a few seconds slowly raise up the body, without giving any jerk to the spine. Take help from the hands, keeping the fingers outward and thumbs towards the belly. Slowly go on raising the back until the whole trunk is at 90^0 and the entire weight comes on the shoulders and neck. Take the legs slightly forward and press the chest with your chin. After remaining in the said pose for a few seconds come to the original position.

Benefits - This asana cures constipation, dyspepsia, has a salutary effect on thyroid gland, tones up the nervous system, all limbs of the body, helps to preserve and thicken semen, is useful in intestinal disorders, varicose veins, appendicitis, renders spine flexible, throat disorders are removed, gas is expelled. In addition, it gives glow, vitality and strength to the body, increases sex power, removes menstrual disorders. Persons with hypertension and cordial problems should never take to this asana, except under advice and guidance and supervision of a yoga teacher.

Chakrasana (A Circle Pose)

Method - On a hard surface, lie flat on your back. Later, raise the middle portion of your body upwards, fixing and keeping firmly both the feet and hands on the ground thus making a semi-circle, ensuring that your head keeps between your hands. Now concentrate your eyes on something that lies in front of you.

Benefits - It enhances, like the sarvanagasana, strength of head, throat, neck, abdomen, legs, hands and, in short, all parts of your body, eliminates pains in joins, removes extra fat from the abdominal area, activates digestive system, renders spinal column elastic and supple, imparts glow and agility to the body, normalises posture and stance, and the body stays erect even during the advanced age. Pregnant ladies should not practice this asana as it can adversely affect their pregnancy process, even leading to miscarriage and bleeding.

Kagasana (The Crow Pose)

Method - This asana can be done three or more times in a day at the rate of 30 seconds per asana or more. Squat on the floor. Keep the arms between your heels and legs, heels being raised on toes. Now, place both the palms flat on the ground (in front), while keeping arms in line and shoulders stretched out as much as possible. Thereafter, raise your body on the toes and endeavour to put pressure on your already spread hands. Remain in this position from ½ to 1 minute and then retrace to the original position and finally relax.

Benefits - This posture helps to diminish the unwanted arches on the spine by helping it to elongate, it strengthens muscles of arms and shoulders, helps to activate hormonal secretions. Old, emaciated and pregnant ladies should resist from doing this asana. Those who have pains in arms, hands and fingers should also abstain, as weak limbs may not be able to withstand weight of the body. This asana should be practised, like many other asanas, on empty stomach only.

Kukkutasana (Cock Pose)

Method - Sit in the position of Padamasna. Insert the hands between the opening to thighs and calves. Now push down the hands and plant them firmly on the floor, keeping your fingers fully spread. Now, after that, push the legs and thighs up your arms. In doing so, your hands turn full so that you could exert desired and sustainable force in lifting the body up. Keep your torso in an upright position, as far as possible. Remain in the final position for a minute or so.

Benefits - Your chest and shoulder muscles become firm due to pressure on them. It also develops and hardens breast-line of females who have small breasts, provided they practise this posture for quite some time.

Mahavirasana (Named After Lord Mahavir/ Hanuman)

Method - Stand erect, bringing forward one foot to a distance of 3 feet from the other. Clench fists of both the hands and raise them. Now, go on jumping alternatively on both the feet, changing the pressure on each feet alternatively. Keep your lips to each other and breathe through nose only. When you are tired, take pause until you regain strength to resume the asana. Loosen your limbs and relax.

Benefits - It increases height, sheds extra weight from the waist, body is rendered stronger, chest expands, legs, arms and feet gain strength. It increases sexual power, especially of men, restores normally to menstrual cycle.

Mayurasana (Peacock Pose)

Method - Stand erect alongside of a table. Place both the hands firmly on top of the table. Fold both elbows in such a way

Important Yogasanas for Everyone

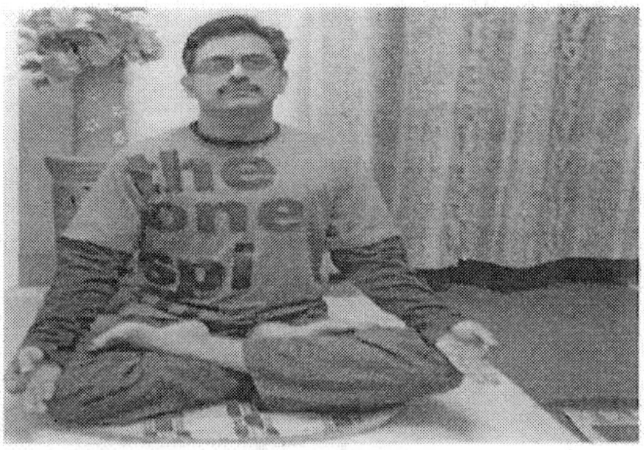

Padmasana

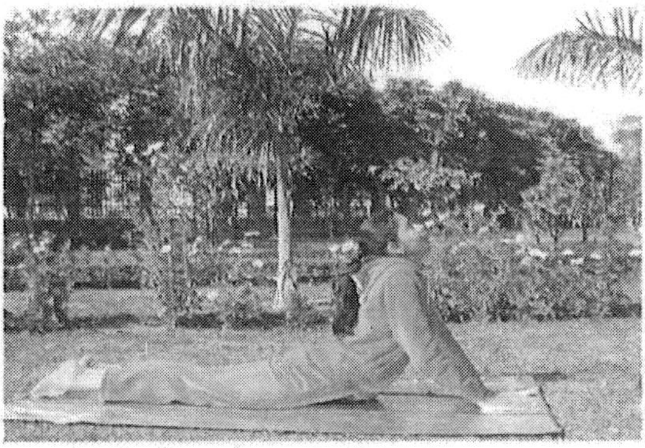

Bhujangasana

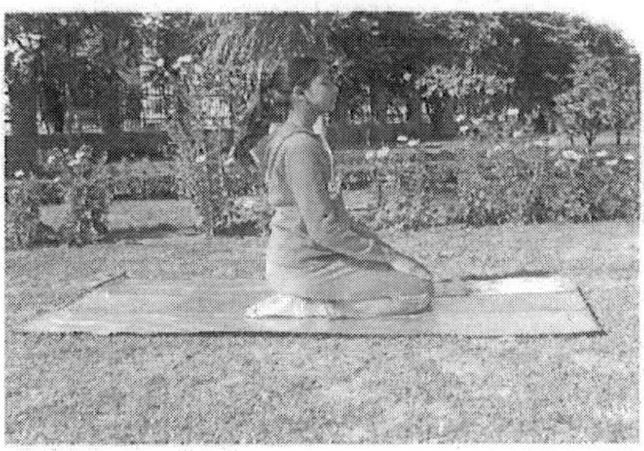

Vajrasana

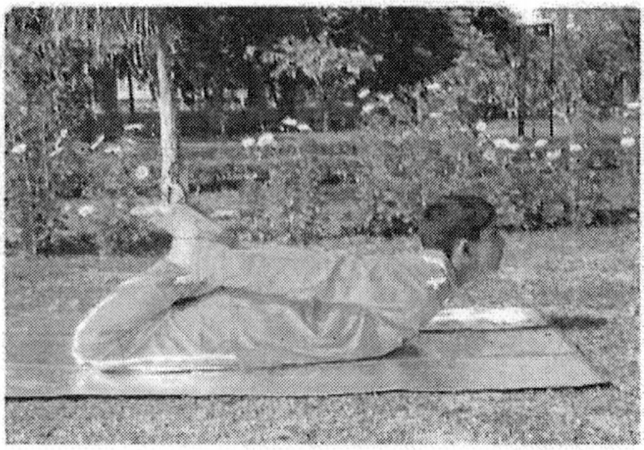

Dhanurasana

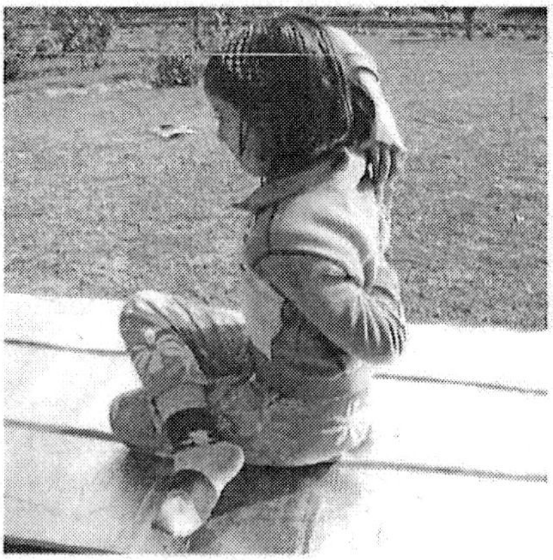

Gomukhasana 1.

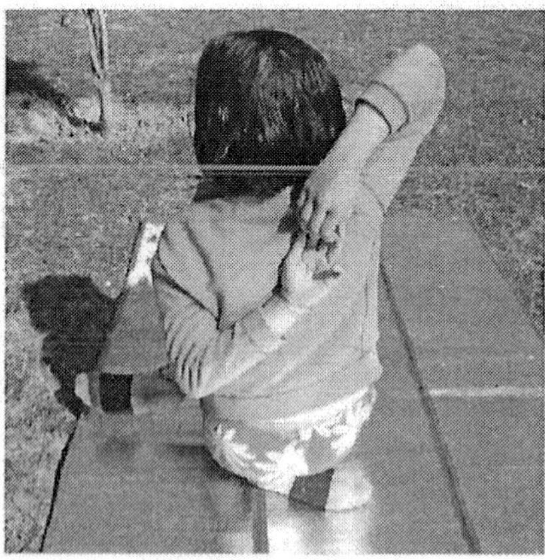

Gomukhasana 2.

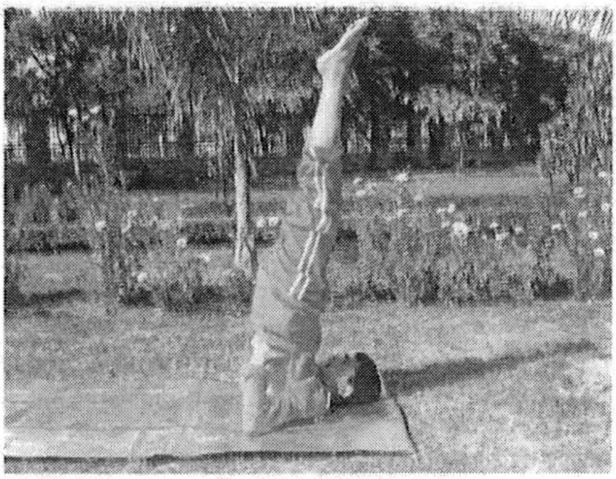

Sarvangasana

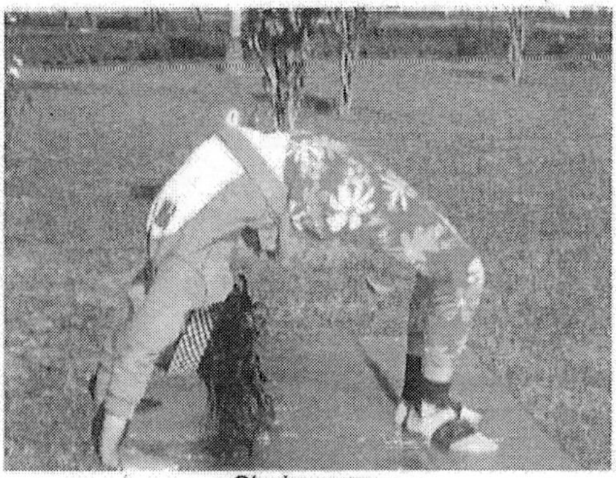

Chakrasana

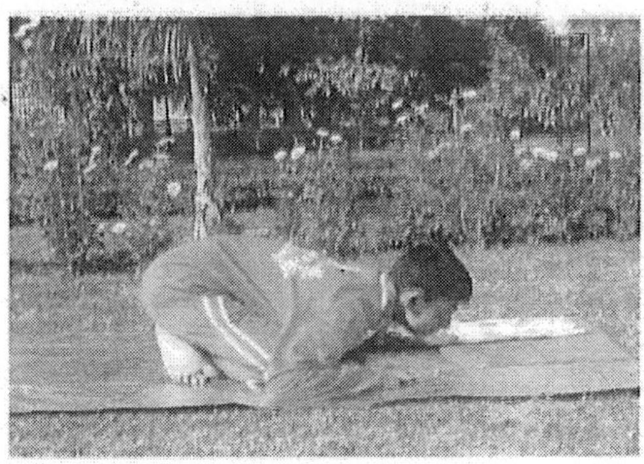

Kagasana

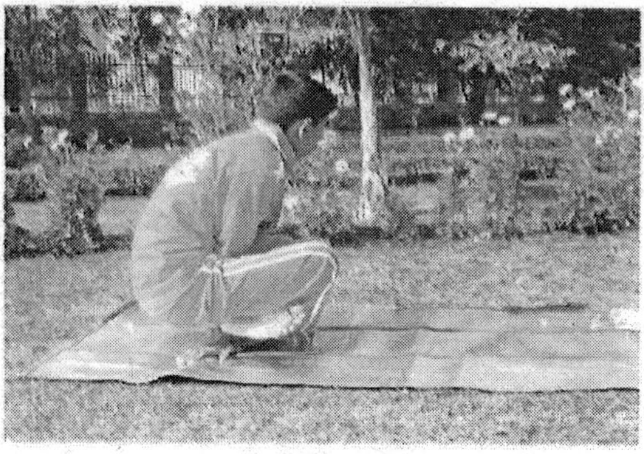

Kukkutasana

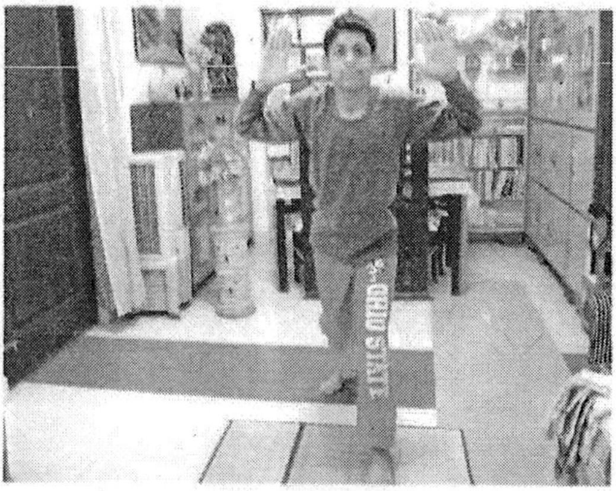

Mahavirasana

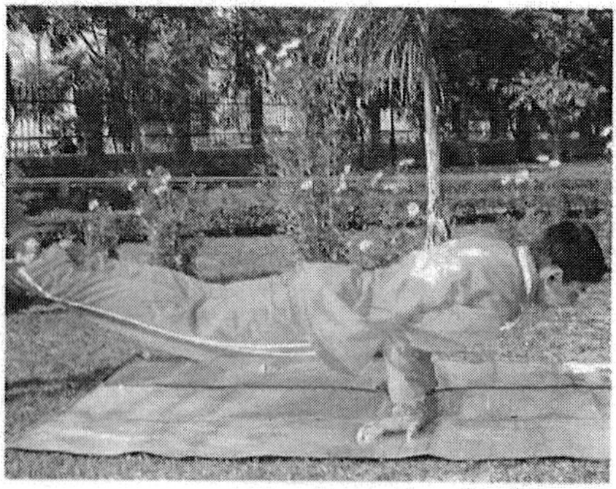

Mayurasana

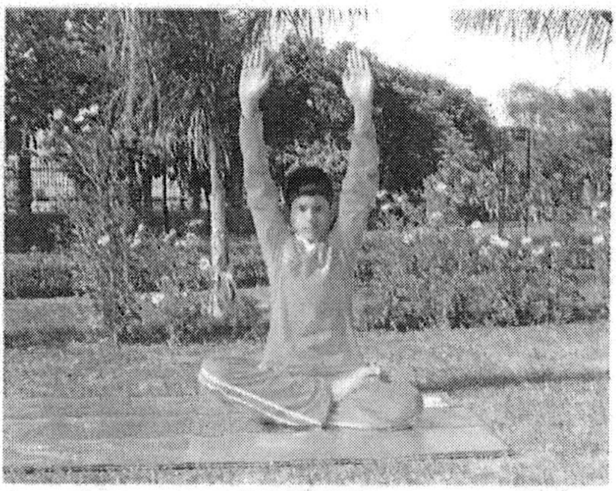

Parvatasana

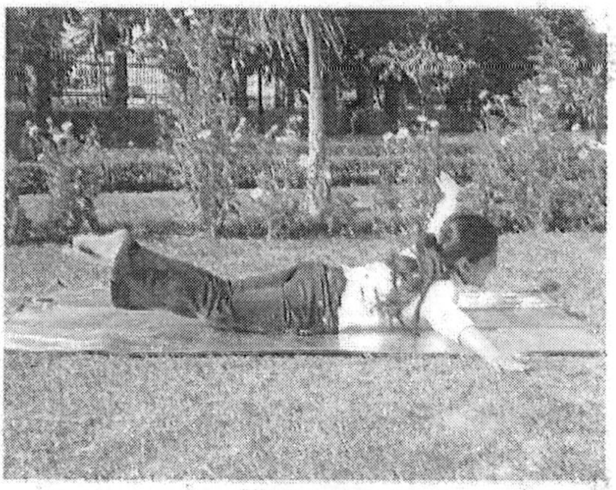

Yanasana

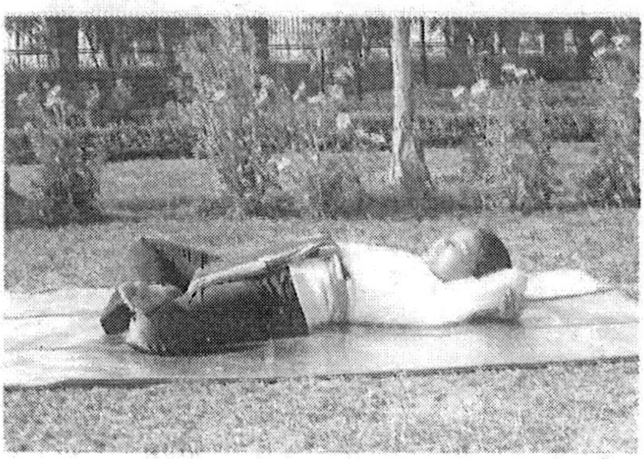

Matsyasana 1.

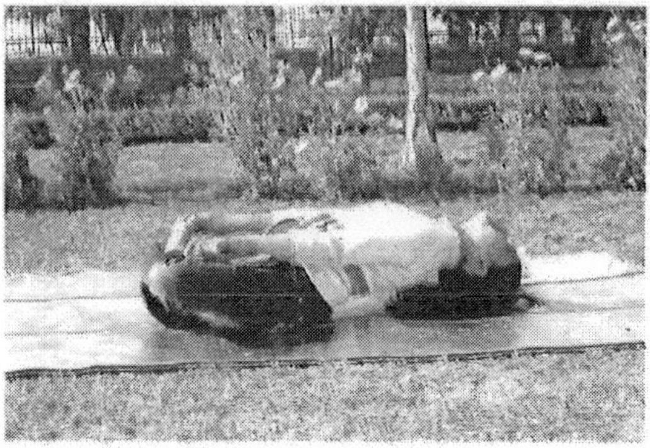

Matsyasana 2.

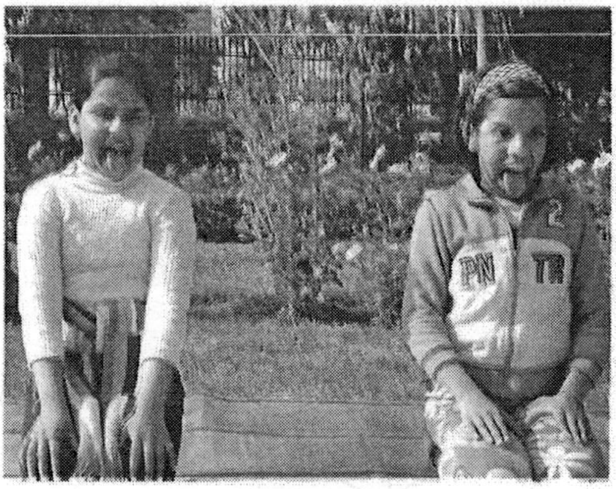

Sinhmudra 1.

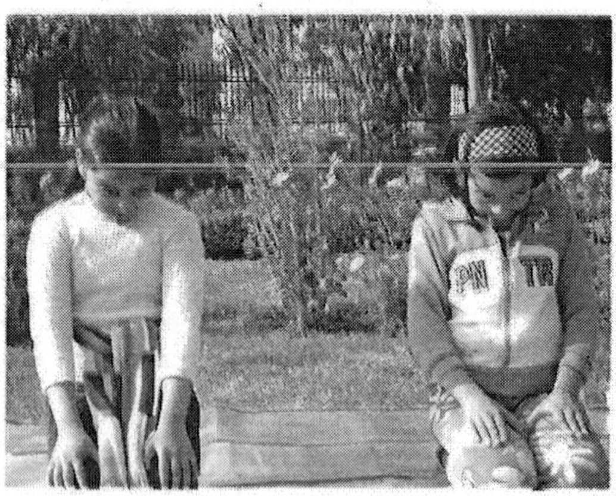

Sinhmudra 2.

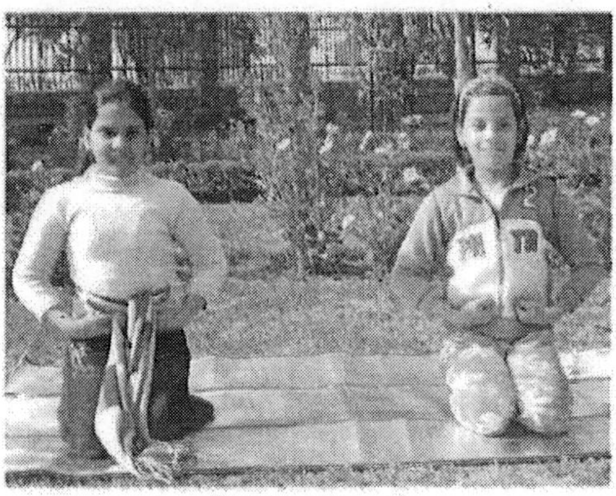

Mandukasana 1.

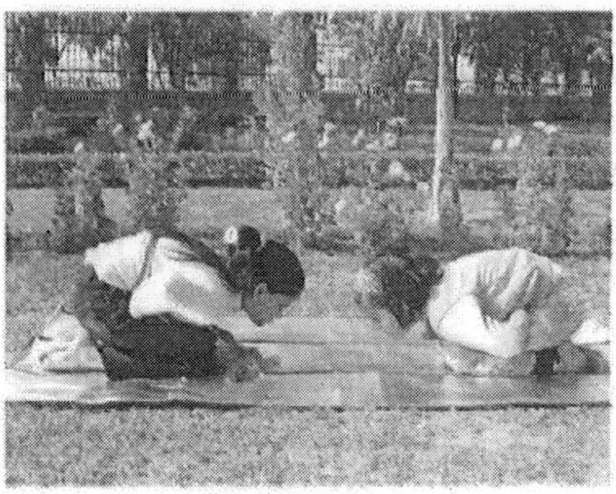

Mandukasana 2.

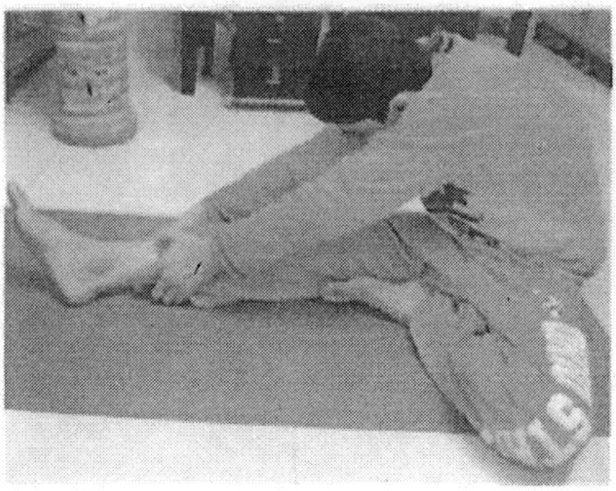

Janushirasana

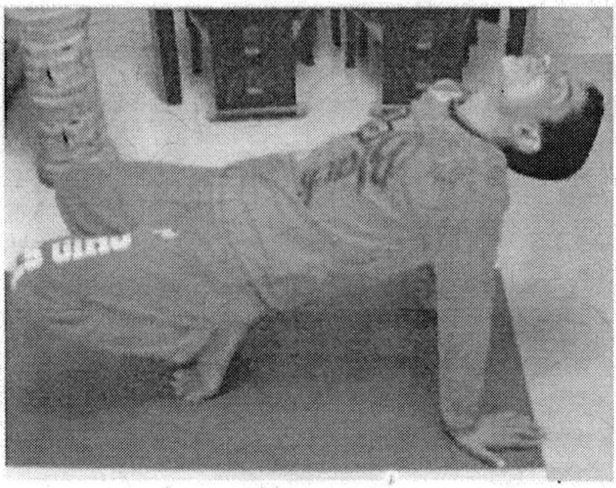

Ushtrasana

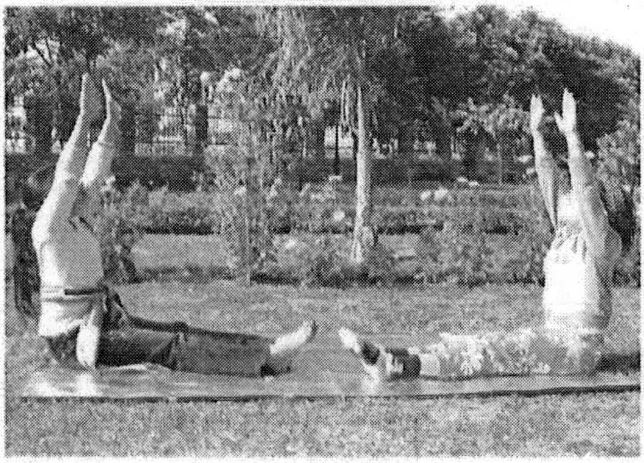

Paschimottanasana 1.

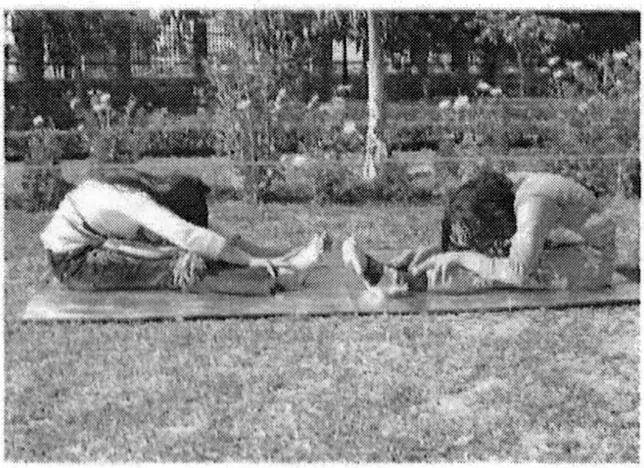

Paschimottanasana 2.

Asanas To Reduce Lethargy Obesity/Diabetes/Thyroid and Other Disorders

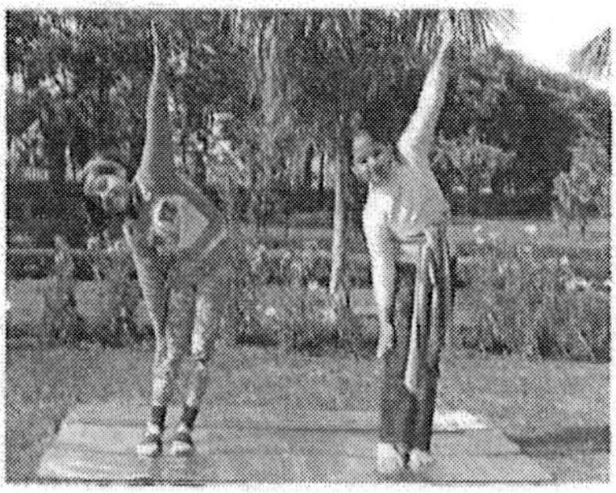

Trikonasana

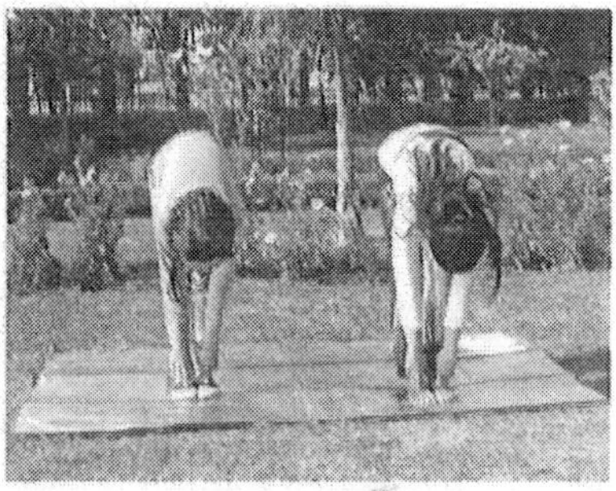

Padhastasana

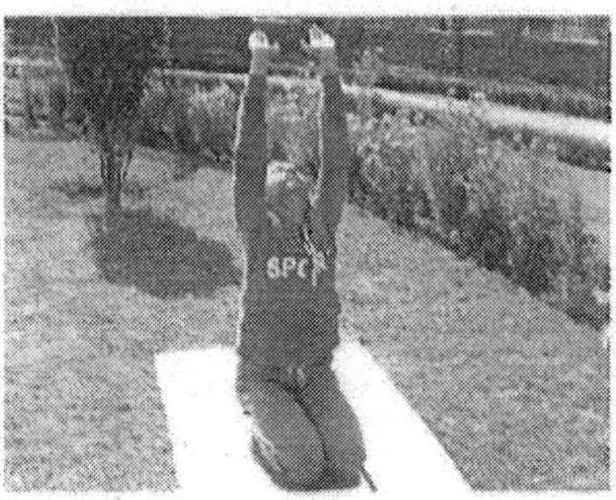

Shashankasana 1.

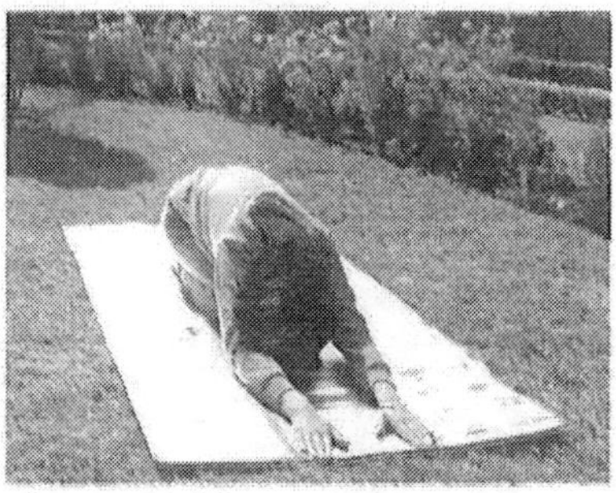

Shashankasana 2.

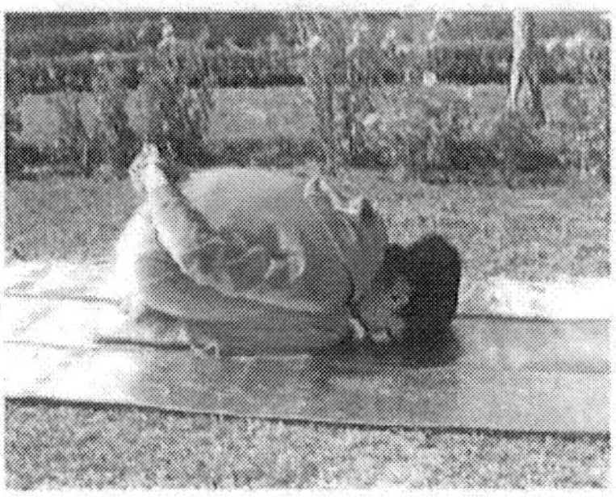

Yogic Exercise for Thyroid 1.

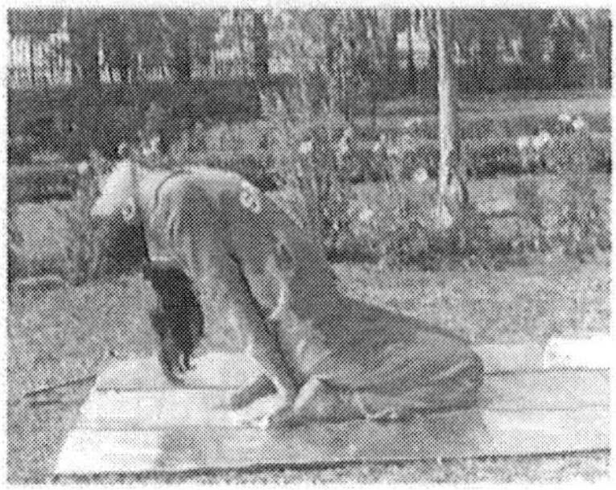

Yogic Exercise for Thyroid 2.

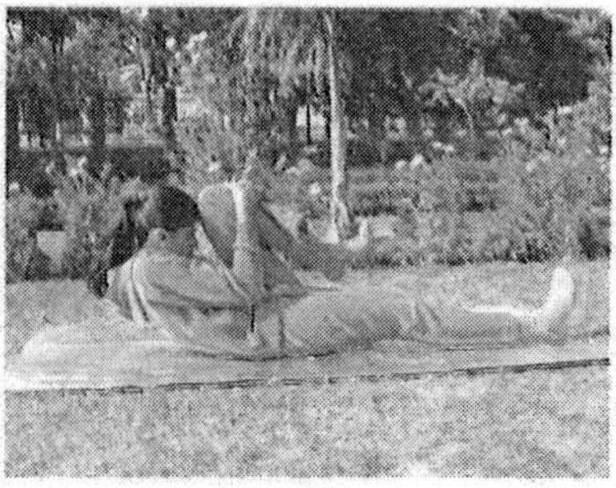

Pawan Muktasana 1.

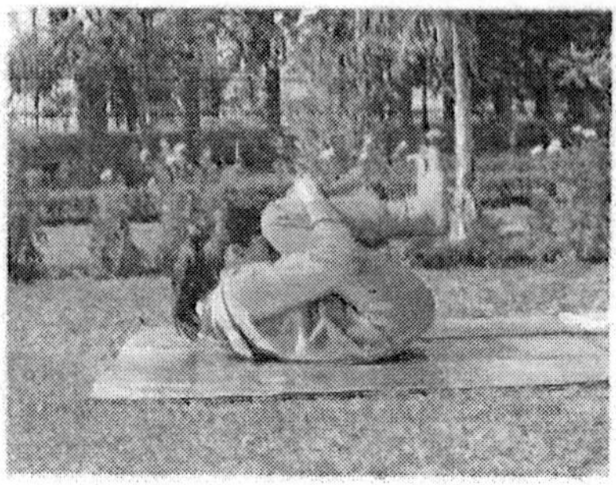

Pawan Muktasana 2.

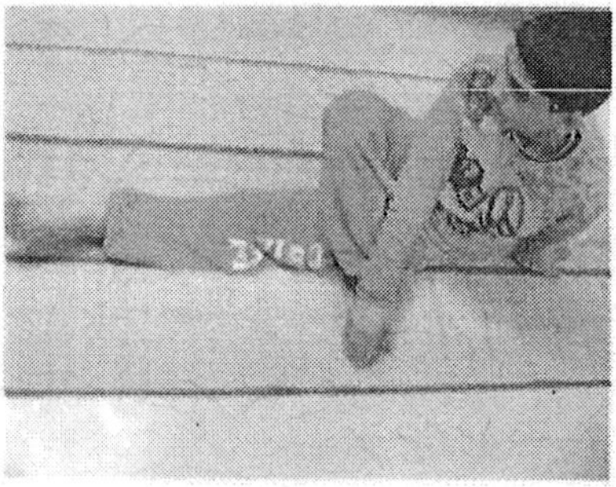

Ardhmatsyandrasana

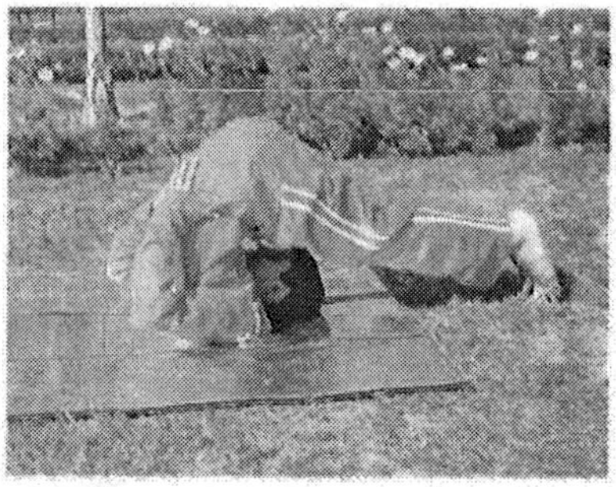

Halasana

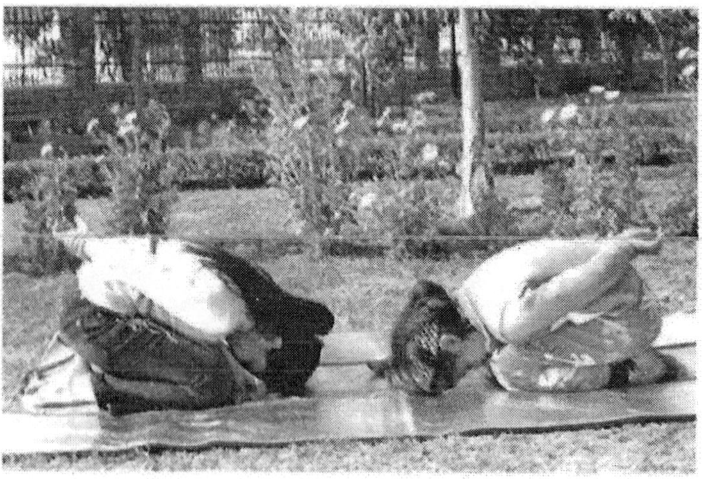

Yoganidra

Asanas to Increase Height, Stretch spine, Eye exercise, Control Digestive System, Hasya Yoga, Acupressure and Others

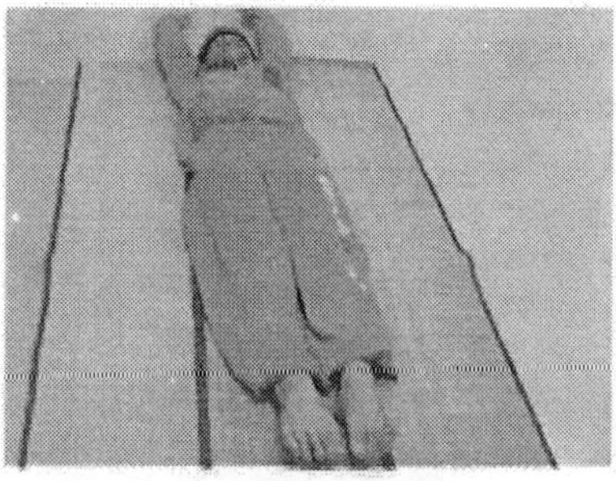

Sarvottanasana
(Stretching the body)

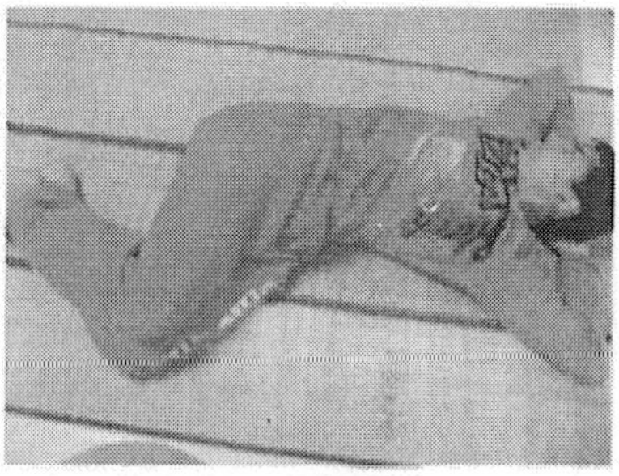

Spinal Stretch 1.

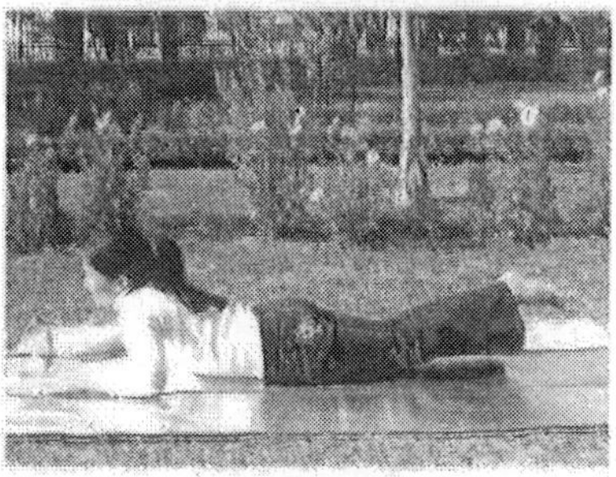

Spinal Stretch 2.

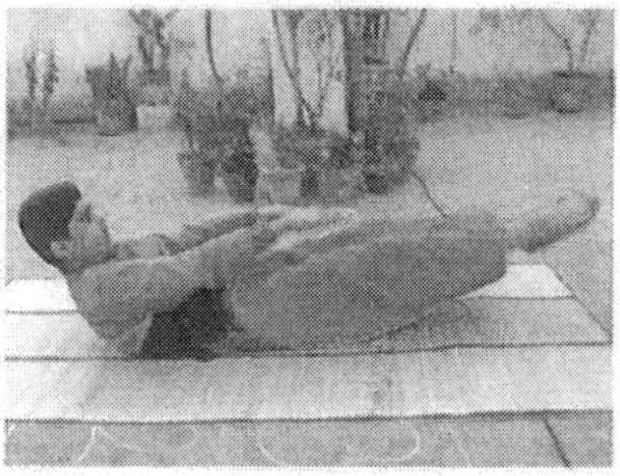

Spinal Stretch 3.

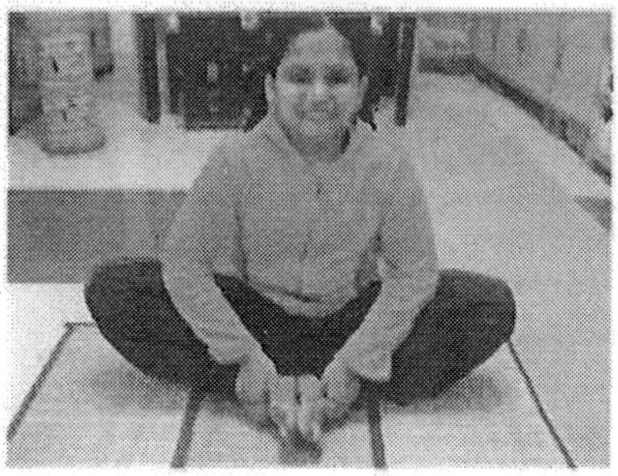

Butterfly

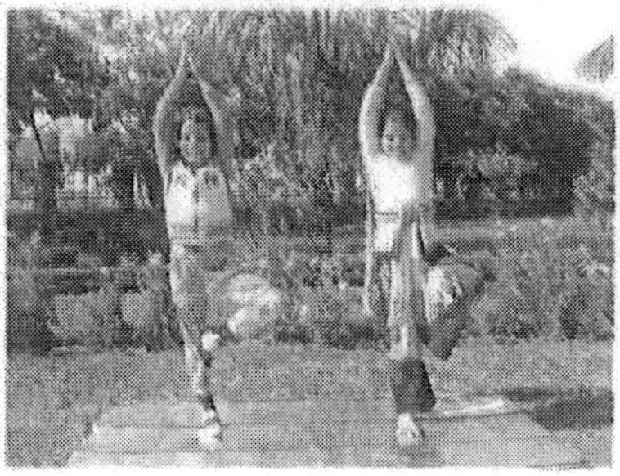

Vrikshasana

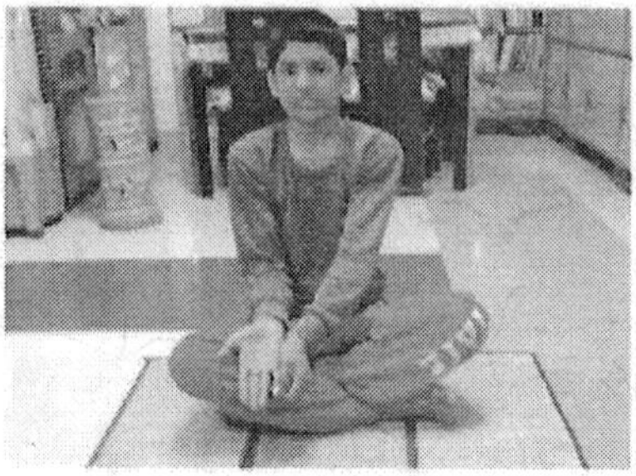

Accupressure Points 1.

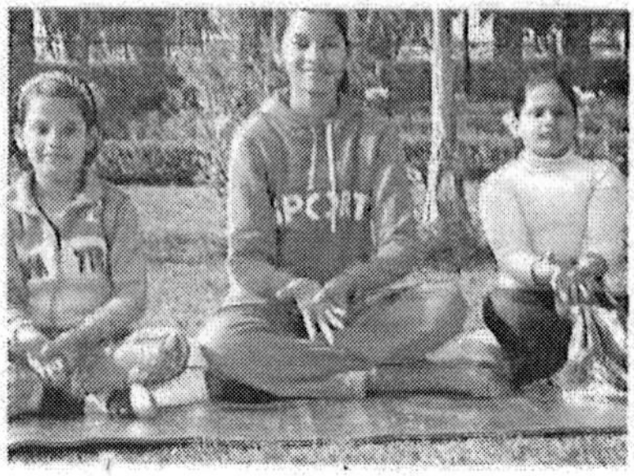

Accupressure Points 2.

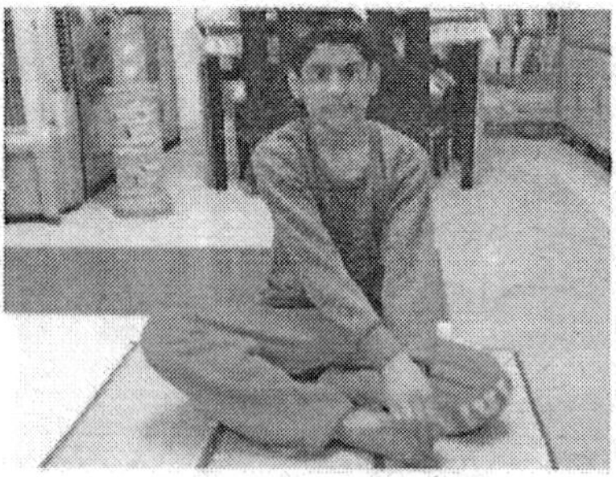

Accupressure Points 3.

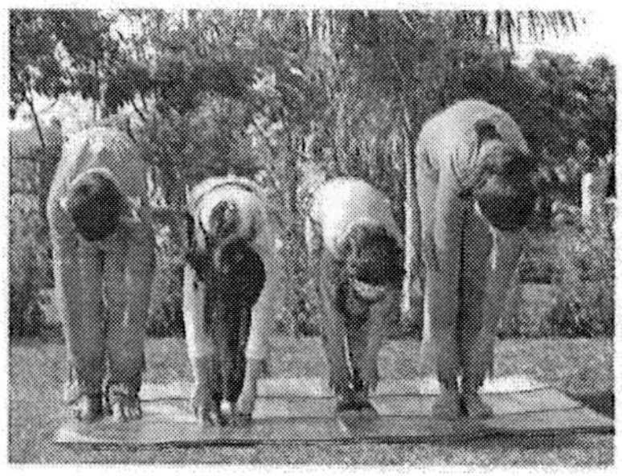

Hasya Yoga 1.

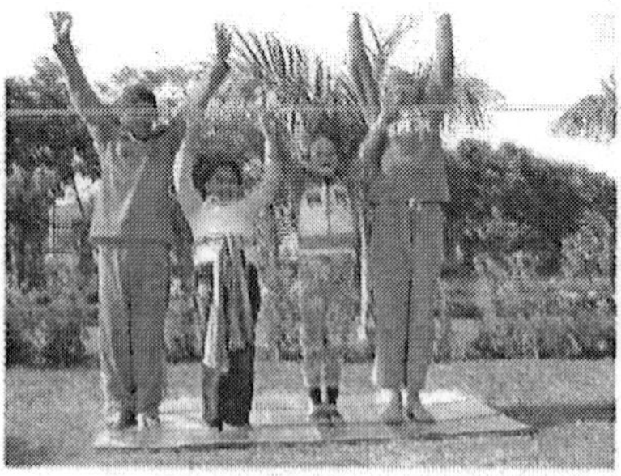

Hasya Yoga 2.

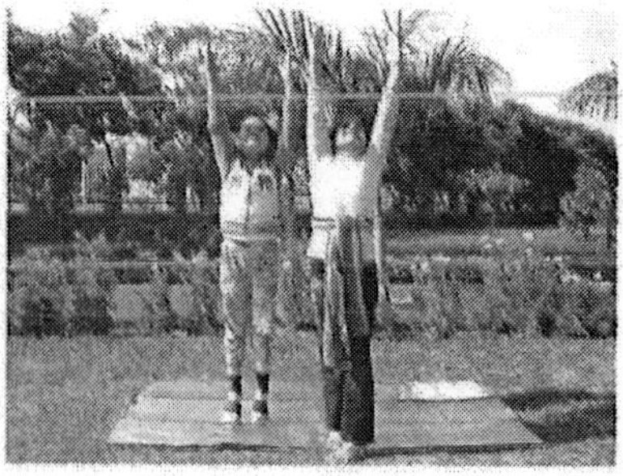

Tarasana 1.

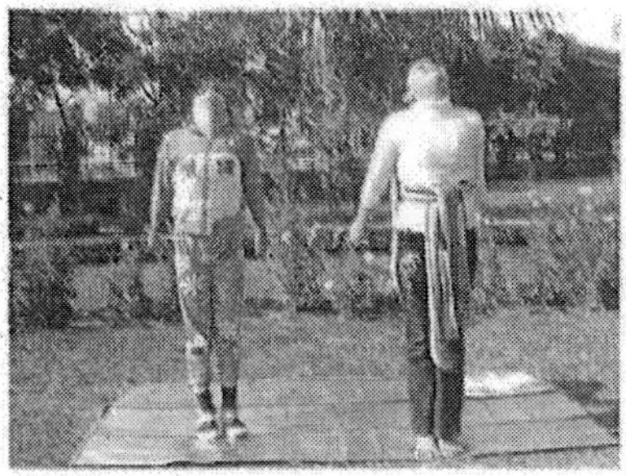

Tarasana 2.

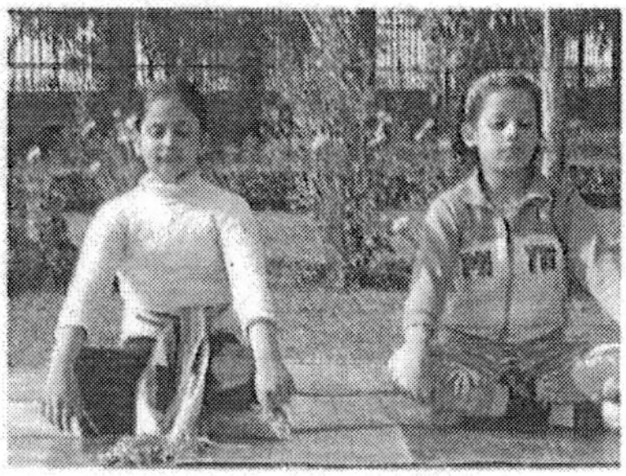

Eye Exercise 1.

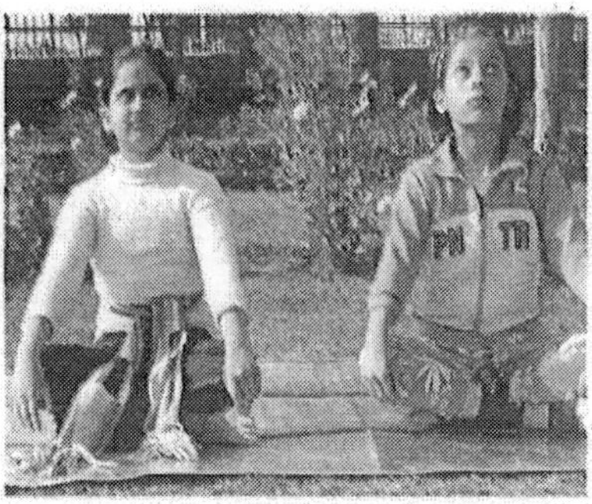

Eye Exercise 2.

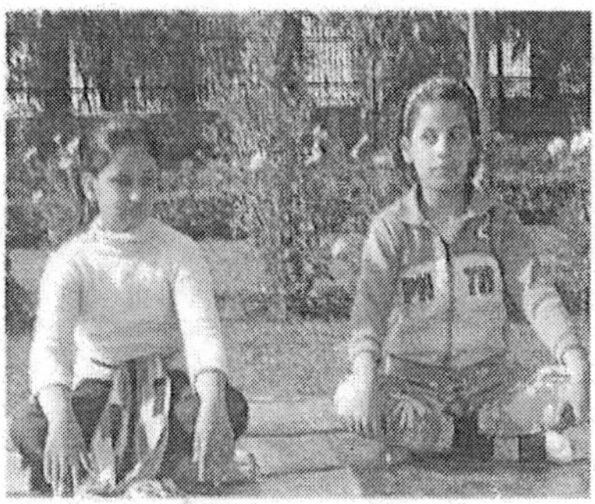

Eye Exercise 3.

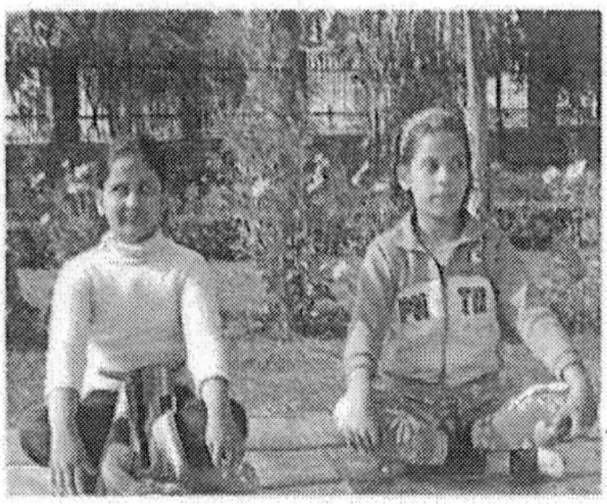

Eye Exercise 4.

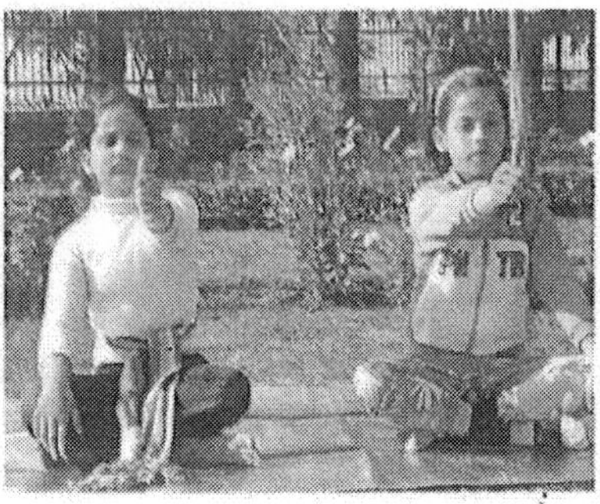

Eye Exercise 5.

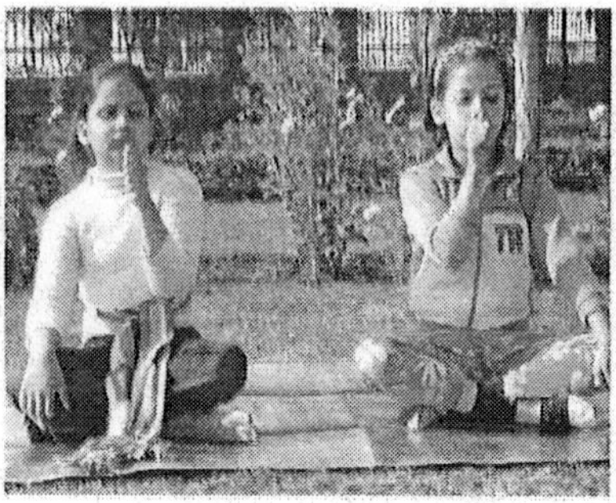

Eye Exercise 6.

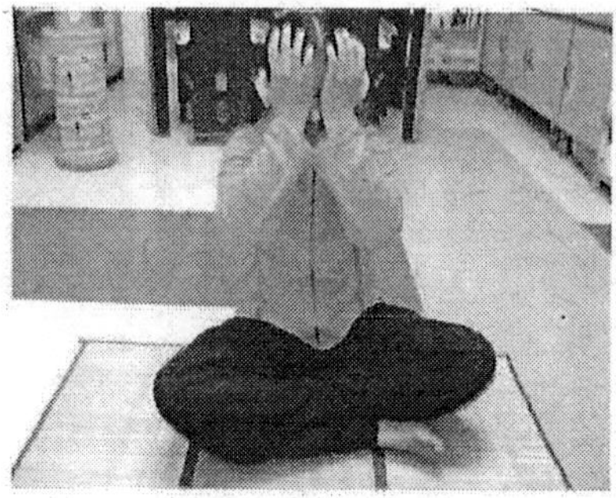

Eye Exercise 7.

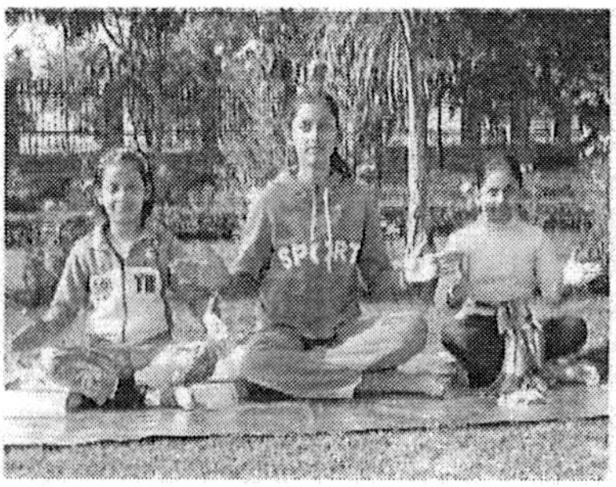

Clapping 1.

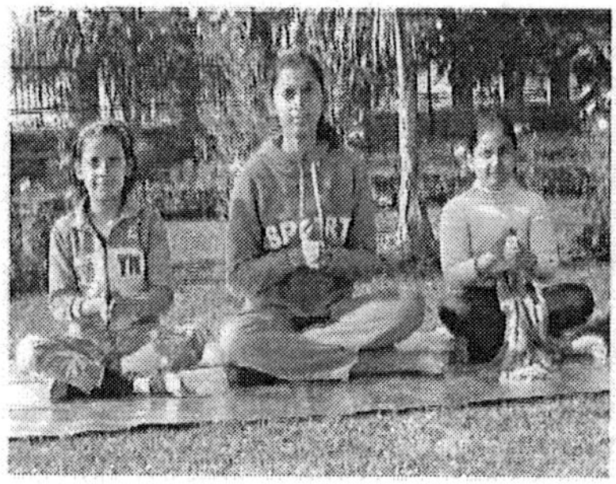

Clapping 2.

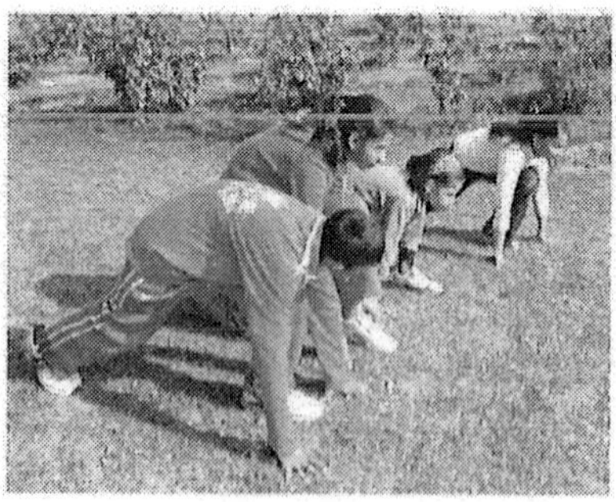

Running 1.

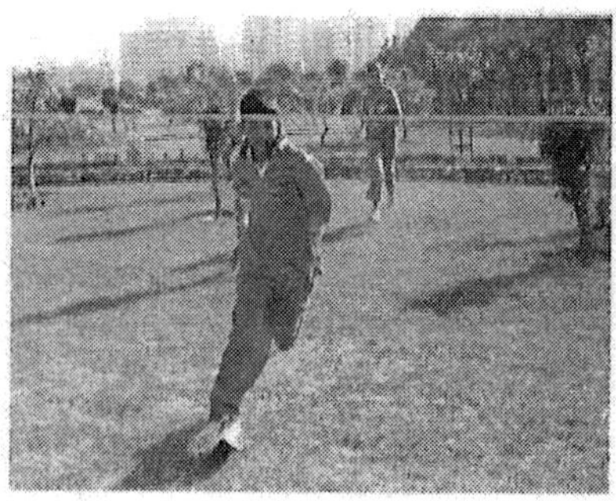

Running 2.

Mudras for Quick Relief

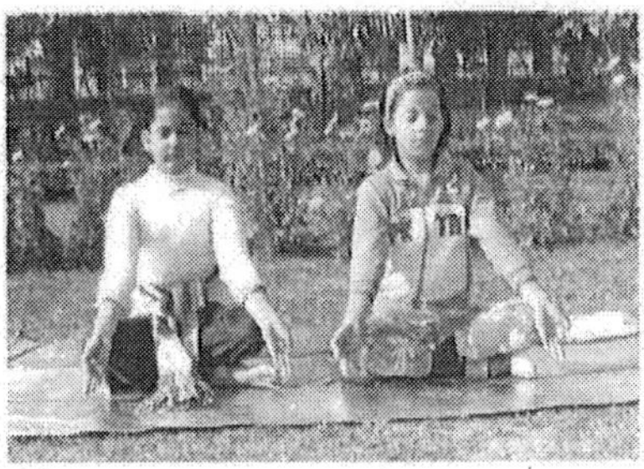

Gyan Mudra

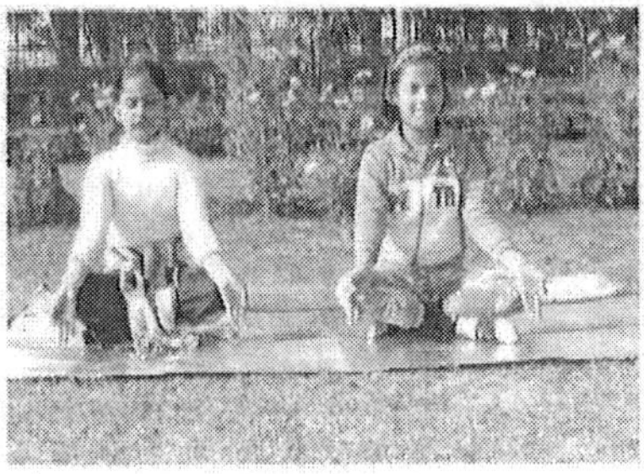

Vairagya Mudra

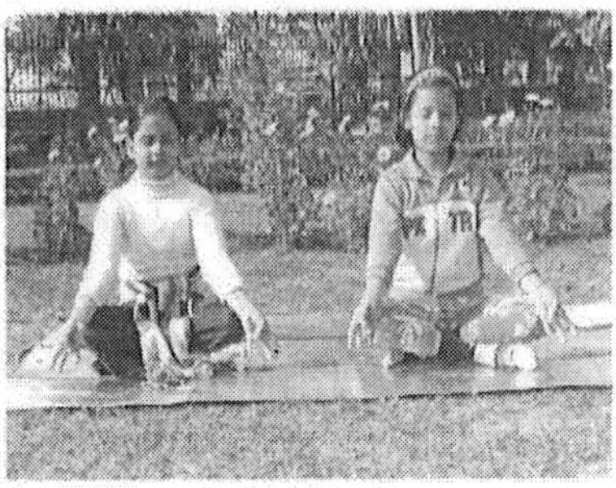

Prithvi Mudra

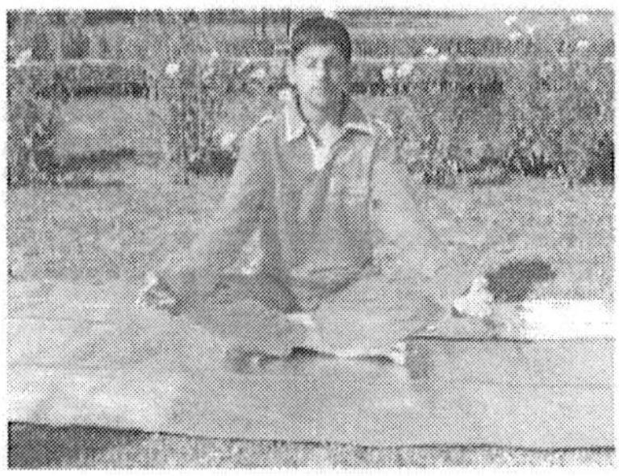

Abhay Mudra

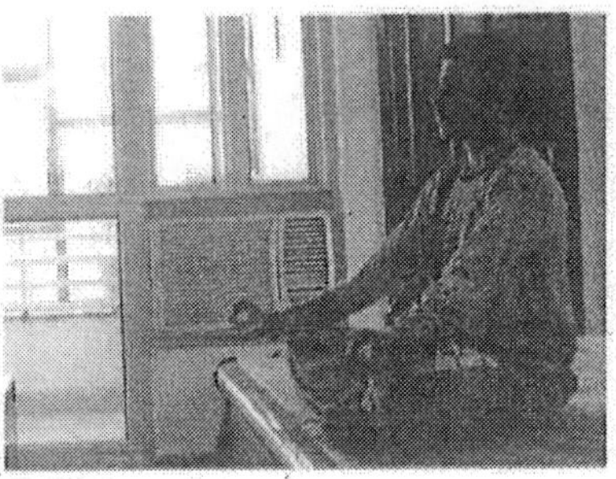

Dhyan Mudra

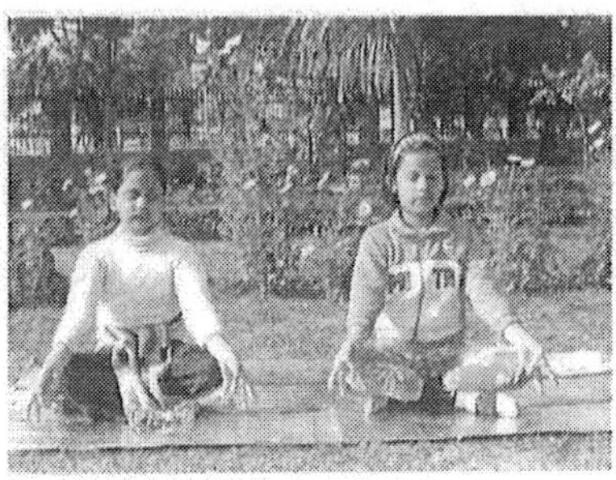

Surya Mudra

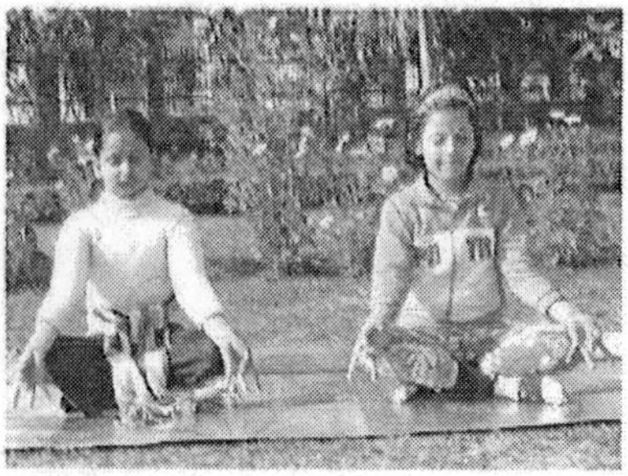

Shoonya Mudra

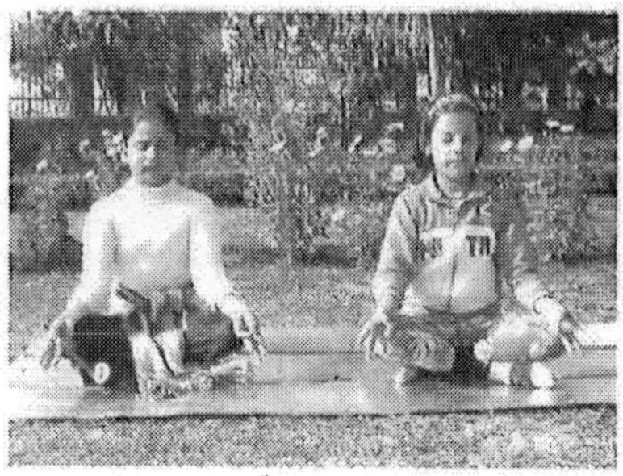

Vayuu Mudra1.

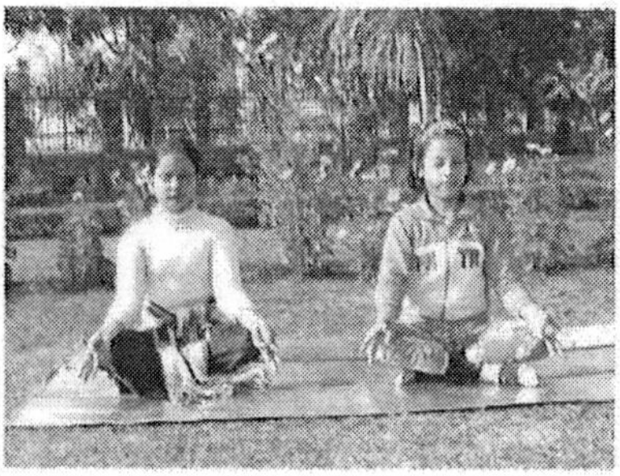

Vayuu Mudra 2.

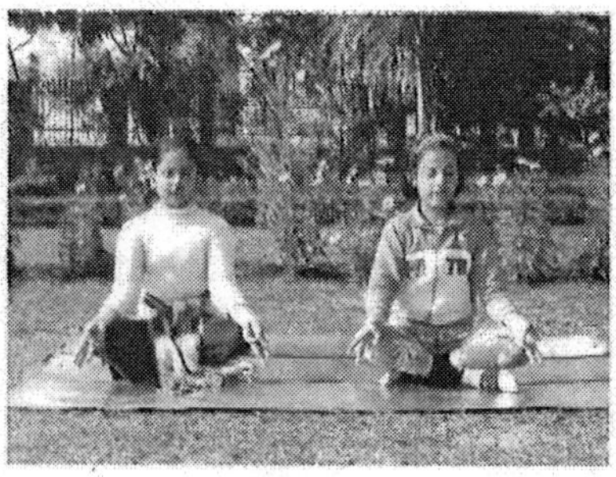

Varun Mudra

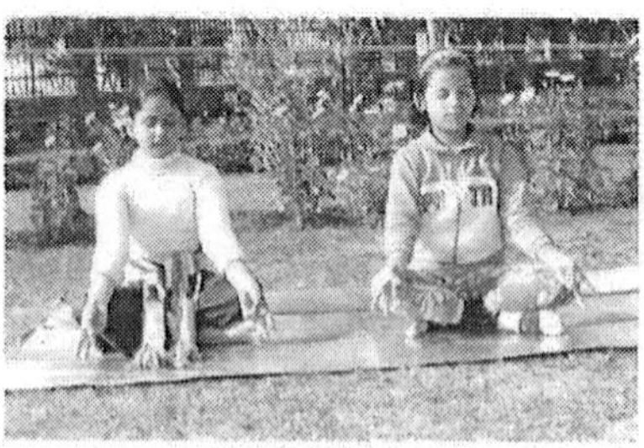

Prana Mudra

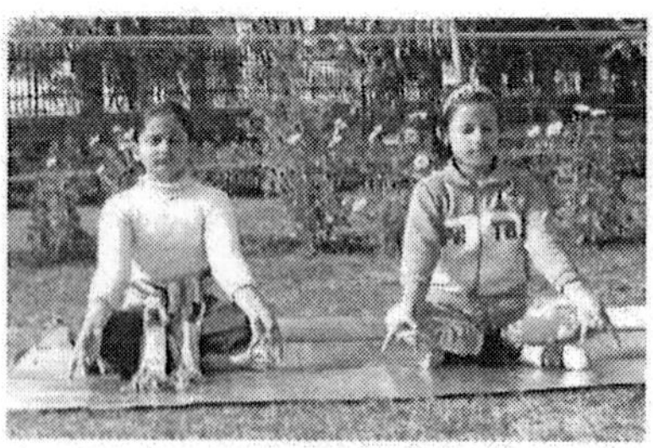

Apaan Mudra

that the elbows touch and remain firmly (touched) near naval. Now, exert whole weight on your hands, by lifting your body at 180^0 and try to stay in this position for 40-50 seconds, increasing the duration gradually or, alternatively, spread some blanket or still better lie flat on ground. Firmly affix your hands on ground, your elbows remaining affixed on either side of navel. Now lift your body and put entire weight of body on the hands. Stay in that position for 40 seconds, gradually increasing the duration, depending on your capacity. After staying in that position, very slowly regain the original position and relax.

Benefits - Increases digestion and appetite. Intestines gain strength, constipation and indigestion are dispelled. Liver and kidney disorders get relieved. Above all, if you have taken poison or poisonous food, it will remove the poison and its effects. It is well known that the snake is eaten by the peacock and its name justifies its utility, as it helps to strengthen the body. Pregnant ladies must not do this asana.

Note - Maximum benefits from the said and other asanas can be derived only when performed properly without exceeding your physical capacity, keeping in view your state of health. To derive optimum benefits, to cure a particular disease or disorder, precision and correctness with which an asana is performed and whether all the relevant procedures have been complied with, are the factors which can ensure utility of an asana.

To start with, proper guidance, or how, what and where of each asana intended to be performed should be guided by a yoga teacher and his guidance sought, if and when some problem is encountered. Never exert undue strain on your body because all asanas cannot be performed by all persons and also all asanas are not required to be done by all. Books on yoga, however precise and meticulous they may be, will only give you an initial motivation in the form of a launching pad only. Without a guru, knowledge gained remains half-baked, hence do not forget what you are expected to do and what not.

Parvatasana

Sit in Padmasana (that is by keeping left foot on the right thigh and right foot on the left thigh). Inhale breath and raise both the hands towards the sky, keeping all the fingers apart and stretching both arms without bending either of them. Stay in the said position as per your capacity and convenience but do not overdo. Before you get suffocated, gradually bring down both the arms and place on both the knees and relax, but without bending your back. Keep spinal column erect at 90^0. The process can be repeated a number of times. In normal conditions ladies can also perform this asana, but never during pregnancy.

This asana imparts flexibility to the spine, strengthens arms, expands chest, and adds to strength of arms and fingers. Improves flexibility of shoulder blades. It improves upon asthmatic condition and tones up uterus.

Yanasana

While performing this asana, body assumes shape and form of a plane flying in the sky; here its nomeclation as such.

Lie flats on the floor, while your abdomen touches the ground. Keep both the feet touching each other. First inhale and then raise your head, neck, hands, chest and feet above the ground, keeping all these organs tight and straight-only your abdomen touching the ground. When you feel you cannot retain the inhaled breath relax and loosen your limbs. After sometime, it can be repeated 3-4 times or even more, if capacity permits. Even while maintaining normal breath, this asana can also be performed. Pregnant women must never perform this asana.

This asana helps to strengthen bones of arms, hands, shoulders, and legs and also imparts flexibility to the spine. If performed regularly, it can add to inches also. It removes extra fat, improves digestion, removes almost all uterine disorders, and keeps the body supple. This asana is not suitable for pregnant ladies.

Stand erect and keep the feet apart at a distance of 6". Now gradually bring down the hands and try to touch the ground in front of your toes. While doing so, exert no pressure nor strain unduly. If initially you cannot touch the ground, it is advisable to bend only to the extent possible. As your back and spine become supple, process will look much easier. Do not bend knees, and elbows, keeping your neck straight at 180^0 while your eyes are affixed looking at the ground or at your hands.

This asana elongates legs and arms, makes spine flexible and supple, improves eyesight, strengthens bones and muscles of legs and hands, and does away with trembling. Persons with backache, hip-joint disease and pregnant ladies must not perform this asana. It also strengths heart, improves cardiac output and efficiency. Improves respiration.

Note: - As a general rule any forward bending asana or any physical exercise should never be performed by persons having stiff back, backache and lumbar /spinal spondylsis/curvature. Backward bending asana/exercise may be performed if advised by the concerned experts.

Matsyâsana (Fish Pose)

Sit in Padmasana and thereafter lie down on your back. Catch hold of big toe of feet with hands and rise up your back portion in a gradual manner. In this position your backside of head and knees should continue to touch the ground. Retain breath as long you can and stay in the final position and exhale while returning to the previous state.

It strengthens chest and lungs, removes extra fat from hips, strengthens legs and hands, dispels asthma, and removes constipation. In normal health conditions ladies can perform this asana, but not during pregnancy.

Pashchimottanasana

Sit on the floor and spread both legs in front of you. Hold each of your big toes with both the hands, but do not let your knees bend. In order to catch the toes you have to bend the back. Initially it may seem slightly difficult to do so, due to rigidity of muscles and limbs; hence do not exert but gradually do the asanas. In 4-5 sittings your body will get attuned to the final posture. Persons with back pain and stiff muscles, pregnant ladies should not perform this asana unless and until advised by a doctor or yoga expert.

It strengthens legs, arms and renders the spine flexible and supple, improve digestion, removes fat on and around abdomen, constipation fortifies and rejuvenates energy and nervous system, lengthens leg bones, purifies blood, improves liver, cardiac and respiratory processes, removes fat from hips and sideways.

Note: - Those who get adept on this asana, may try to touch their knees with the nose but in the changed position also knees shouldn't be bent.

Janushirasana

Sit on the floor and fold leg from the knee and place heel of left leg below the anus. Keeping the other leg straight. Catch hold of the right foot and try to touch the knee of the spread out leg with your nose/ mouth. There won't be any difficulty if you can perform the 'Pashchimottana Asana'. Return to normal position. Now repeat the same process with the right leg. When done, relax. You may fully succeed after 5-6 attempts and until a successful posture is achieved never exert undue pressure. Pregnant ladies, backache persons who have stiff spine, muscles and joints, should not perform it, but others may proceed gradually in a phased manner.

Ushtrasana

This asana has been named after the camel. Sit erect and let the weight of entire body fall on both knees and toes of feet. Now catch hold of your heels with the hands. While performing this asana, make sure that the back is bent in such a way that neck bends towards feet, back also bends slightly. Look upwards. Stay in the final position as far and as you conveniently can. Retain breath and exhale while getting back to the original (starting) position.

This asana strengthens back, spine, knees, and feet renders spine flexible. After the asana is over, there may be felt ache and stiffness in shoulder blades, knees and feet. To ward off all such effects massage these parts with coconut or mustard oil. This asana is capable of increasing height. Pregnant ladies shouldn't perform this asana as it exerts utmost pressure on abdomen and back, but in normal health condition, they may perform this asana, especially when they have backache. Avoid undue pressure and jerk in any case.

Sinhamudra

Yogic exercises should accompany breathing in rhythm only through the nostrils. This asana is an exception where one cannot do so, because the tongue has to be folded and then stretched in two stages.

Method - Kneel down and lower the body to sit on heels as in Vajrasana except that in Vajrasana the Knees are kept close together and in this they are kept slightly apart. Spread both the palms and place them on the knees in a relaxed way. Breathe evenly, protrude the tongue and fold inwards to touch the palate. Bend the head a little forward, the chin touching the chest. At the same time exhale through the nose as well as the mouth simultaneously stretching the tongue as much as possible out of the mouth. Widen the eyes and fix the gaze in front. Remain thus for two-three seconds and not more during the initial days. Once the protrusion of the tongue is completed, you should stop exhaling and hold the breath for two seconds. After two seconds, slowly draw in the tongue and inhale only through the nose and sit erect. Repeat the process again. After a few days of practice, this exercise can be perfected and practised as many times as possible.

Benefits - This exercise is extremely useful to all young children and must be practised by adults to prevent and cure a number of diseases connected with ear, nose, throat and other respiratory troubles.

It helps greatly in overcoming all problems related to tonsils, adenoids, larynx and pharynx. If regularly practised, it can prevent any unnecessary removal of tonsils by surgery. As the face and eye muscles are exercised, it gives a glowing colour to the complexion and shine to the eyes. This exercise proves to be extremely beneficial to singers and public speakers. It is useful in all forms of skin diseases. It cures thyroid diseases and deafness if practised perfectly and regularly.

Mandukasana

This asana must have derived its name for the Sanskrit name Manduka which means a frog. Mandukasana does not resemble the frog very much as its name denotes, but the folded legs resemble frog's hind legs and the arms supporting the body look like frog's forelegs. Though this asana looks simple and is also easy to perform, its benefits are plenty.

Method - Kneel down with the knees apart. Slowly lower the body and sit down between the folded legs in such a way that the buttocks touch the ground. Slowly widen the gap between the knees till they come in a straight line. Keep the toes close to each other. Lean a little forward and place both the palms near the thighs, fingers turned towards the thighs. Keep the spine erect, fix your gaze straight and breath normally. Stay so for as long as you can and revert back to original position by releasing the hands first and then drawing in the folded legs together.

Relax and repeat again.

During the initial days of practice, difficulty may be experienced in spreading the legs and it may not come in straight line. The groins may ache if you force it. Gradually, the gap can be decreased without any discomfort.

Benefits - This is a unique exercises for women, teenage girls as well as women of other ages. All uttering disorders respond well to this exercise. The so-called premenstrual syndrome, like depression, frustration and anxiety can be overcome by practising this asana regularly. It cures impotence in the males. It strengthens the pelvic muscles and improves circulation in the region. It helps control bladder and prostate disorders. Spinal nerves get adequate supply of circulation and they become stronger. It is a good exercise for obesity too.

□□□□

7.
ASANAS TO REDUCE OBESITY, DIABETES, THYROID AND OTHER DISORDERS

Here are some other important yogasanas which help in controlling diabetes, thyroid problems, spinal curves and obesity, laziness and improving concentration .

Trikonasana

Stand straight with legs a bit apart. Then inhale deeply and while exhaling bend towards your left, keeping spine straight. Then repeat in the opposite side.

It is very good to improve the lethargy and laziness and increases energy level. It also vanishes energy acidosis and improves circulation in whole body. It is also helpful in treating the intoxication.

Padhastasana

Stand straight and inhale deeply. Keep both hands up. Then bend forward exhaling to touch your toes by fingers and try to touch your nose with knees.

It is good to reduce extra fat on abdomen, stretches the spinal chord and relaxes the muscles of spinal cord.

Shashankasana

Sit in vajrasana (described separately). Then inhale deeply and lift your both hands up, keeping the spine straight. Then while exhaling bend forward from the waist and try to touch the elbows, hands and palms to ground and slowly the forehead also.

It is helpful in improving digestive system, reduces obesity and is also good for the female reproductive system.

Thyroid Controlling Asana

Sit in vajrasana pose. Now bend both hands on back and hold one wrist from other hands palm. While exhaling bend your waist forward and touch your forehead on ground.Now keep tied hands up facing sky. Now while inhaling, turn straight and put your hands on ankles and try to keep your chest and abdomen straight and bend your neck to back and look at the sky.

It is one of the best yogasanas for thyroid gland and metabolic reactions in body.It is also good for correcting the bent spine and helps in keeping the bent posture proper.

Yoganidra

Sit in vajrasana pose.Bend your hand back and hold wrist of one hand from the other hand. Now inhale deeply and while exhaling bend forward and try to touch the forehead to the ground. Remain for thirty seconds to one minute in this pose.

It is good for stubborn kids and helps in improving the behaviour. It is good for concentration also. It relaxes the mental anxities.

□□□□

8.
ASANAS TO INCREASE HEIGHT, STRETCH SPINE, EYE EXERCISES, CONTROL DIGESTIVE SYSTEM, HASYA YOGA, ACUPRESSURE AND OTHERS

To develop life force, here are some easy exercises which you can learn easily :-

Sarvottanasana (Stretching Pose)

Lie down flat on your back on the carpet. Keep the heels and big toes of both the feet close together. Interlock the fingers of both hands and put them on your belly. Now inhaling raise the arms straight above your head so that the hands touch the ground. Stretch pointing the feet forward and arms away from the body and tighten all the muscles of your body. Now inhaling bring the interlocked hand back on the belly and relax for few seconds.Repeat this exercise three times. Relax in Shavasana for fifteen seconds.

Then put you arms sidewise or below head to your body, keeping them little away from your body with palms upwards. Drop the feet sidewise with the big toes pointing in outward direction , keepeng the heels a few inches apart from each other. Similarily rotate left shoulder bone.Kepeat it for 30 times.

Benefits - This practice removes congestion in chest and shoulders.It has very good effect on liver, spleen and eyes. Thyroid and parathyroid glands are also rejuvenated. It is good for joint movement also.

You should also move your feet side by side in the same way.

Butterfly

Sit in sukhasana. Now stretch your legs horizontally to fix the soles of both the feet. Start moving up and down the knees and keep your hands on ankles.

Benefits:- This is a very good exercise for the chakras,especially muladhar.This exercise keeps the level of sex hormones proper so your pleasure and strength increases.

Acupressure Exercises

Acupressure is a great way of keeping life force active and relieving pain. For details, kindly go through the book on Acupressure from the same author,published by the same publisher.

Here in photos, you can see that how to do accu-massage on palms.This increases the flow of channels.You should also pressurise your tips of all fingers with the help of other hand. The tips of feet and soles should also be accu -massaged . This technique increase the flow of energy and sharpens the mind.

There are certain points on ears also. So in early morning while doing exercises, one should also stretch the ears–ear lobes, middle and upper part should be stretched 3-4 times. Clapping is also good.

Hasya Yoga

Laughter is the best therapy to burst the tension and relieve the stress. During laughing our 32 muscles are stretched, so this is an exercise for face also.Try to smile all through the day, as this pose helps in keeping away the negative energies also.Look at the smile of a child,which is innocent smile. Your productivity of work will certainly increase with smile and laughter.

Spinal Stretch

Lie down on abdomen on a mat. Lift your legs and hands as shown in photos.These poses are good for those who have spinal pain, spondylitis in past.During pain do not do this exercise.But otherwise do it regularly to get rid of further pain as this pose stretches the back. The spinal chord is surrounded by nerves and thus the nerves are also re-charged.

Height Increasing Poses

Tarasana and Vrikshasana are one of the best yogic exercises to increase height among children.These are very simple exercises as you can see in photos. In Tarasana you have to stretch your body in standing pose .You should be on your upper part of soles and your palms and fingers of hands should also be stretched towards sky. Stretch your body as much as you can. Look at the second photo also.

This should be practised from the early age of life. Children should also be encouraged to hang on iron rods and play basketball like games to increase height. Running in early morning is also good.

Eye Exercises

Eyes are important organ of body. Eyes exercise should also be done along with other body exercises. Eyes should be rotated in clockwise, anticlockwise direction.Then do the exercise of bringing thumb near eye and taking away. Lastly do the palming of eyes also as shown .

□□□□

9. MUDRAS FOR QUICK RELIEF

Proper Mudras help in proper healing through yoga.

Gyan Mudra

In Yoga Shastra this Mudra is signified as the 'Gyan Mudra'. Here top of index finger is touched with top portion of the thumb, and our saints/yogis have immensely practised on this mudra.

Lord Buddha and Lord Mahavira have been shown in this mudra. In the battle field of Kurukshetra Lord Krishna explained the intricacies of *Geeta* to Arjun in the same Mudra hence its utmost importance.

Thumb signifies Fire element and the index finger represents/signifies Air element. When both the elements conjoin, Gyan Mudra comes into existence and Air element gets established and balanced. By continuous practice of this Mudra, malfunction of symptoms-blood vessels of the brain can be set in order, without aid of any medicine. In addition, irregular and disturbed sleep, weak memory, anger, insanity can be easily dispelled. It also enhances receptive capability whereby a person is able to acquire and store knowledge all around him, in his brain. Persons, whose mental activity has been weakened, should regularly practise this mudra. This mudra is an attribute of Yogic meditation or trance (Samadhi), and is practised to concentrate. Its regular practice fortifies and strengthens nerves.

Vairagya Mudra

Sit in Padmasan, Siddhasana or in any comfortable asana, whichever suits you best. Place both the hands, as was done in Gyan Mudra, on your knees in an upward position, and sit quietly and peacefully. This mudra is formed by touching frontal portion of the thumb with index finger's frontal portion. Swami Dayanad spent major part of his time by sitting in this posture. Most of his devotees are seen sitting in this posture while they have to chanta mantra. After 'Gyan' 'Vairagya' (renunciation) is the next step. Hence Vairagaya and Gyan mudras are practised in unison. This mudra inculcates and develops spirituality and imparts self-knowledge. The devotee becomes mentally and physically healthy, and his spiritual knowledge is also added.

Abhaya Mudra

The practitioner should form Gyan Mudra with both of his hands, and place his hands alongside the shoulders as shown in the picture. As the name of this mudra indicates, it inculcates courage and solid determination in a person. 'Gyan' is followed by 'Vairagya' and self-confidence is the natural outcome of complete knowledge. If practised regularly, it will bring a permanent benefit to a devotee's mind, brain and heart; and he will be relieved permanently from the mental tension and agony. The bigger achievement through this mudra being that a person will not get horrified by fear or any sort of calamity. In ancient times the sages and ascetics used to practise sadhana in the forests. This mudra kept them free from the fear of fierce animals and other problems and, thus, they used to feel courageous and bold.

Dhyana Mudra

To make a pose for Dhyana Mudra a person should place his hands in the same position as are placed in Gyan Mudra that is frontal portion of his thumb and index finger should touch with each other and then he should place the same upon his laps, while sitting in any comfortable posture. This mudra also helps in concentration of the mind, because, as the mudras explained earlier, base of this mudra is also the Gyan Mudra. Dhyana Mudra, if practised regularly for a longer span of time, imparts a unique and divine bliss. It is also very useful for mental agony and agitation. In addition, it also keeps blood pressure under control.

Vaayu Mudra

Turn the index finger and touch it with the base (root) of the thumb, exerting very light pressure. Index finger controls air element (one of the five elements) and any imbalance in air element can emerge in the form of wind related diseases. Vaayu Mudra effectively treats many wind related incurable diseases like gout, polio, paralysis, trembling or Parkinson's diseases and acts as a medicine.

Shoonya Mudra

If the middle finger's tip is touched at the root (base of the thumb as shown in the picture) it forms Shoonya mudra.

Shoonya represents sky (or vacuum) element, and is synonym of the sky. Sky element is present even in a minute object of this universe, apart from it the same element is present in every part of our body. When this element gets disbalanced, many diseases surface. Vaccum element is directly related to sound, hence due to its disbalance, many ear related diseases ensue. When there is a pain in the ear, it can be subsided quickly if this mudra is practised at the inception stage of pain and thus, many ear related problems like discharges from the ear, chronic ear ache, deafness and hard of hearing can be cured effectively, if this mudra is practised for 45 minutes daily.

Surya Mudra

As the name indicates, it is a brilliant mudra. Join or touch your ring finger (anamika) at the root of thumb (as shown in the picture) maintaining light pressure. Ring finger represents earth element, and the thumb represents fire element. According to *Saamudrik Shastra,* ring finger is the seat of the sun. Hence, when ring finger is pressed at the root of the thumb, plenty of energy is generated which can and should be compared with solar energy.

Surya Mudra is particularly effective in curing any type of headache or sense of heaviness in the brain. It also resolves problem of obesity.

Varun Mudra

Varun Mudra is formed by joining the little finger's top with the top of the thumb. The little finger represents water element. By continuous practice of this mudra, all the diseases that are caused by lassitude of water element, can be treated. It also imparts glow and smoothness to the face.

It also removes roughness from the face, apart from removing facial wrinkles and purifying the blood. It also restores elegance and cleanliness to the face.

Prithvi Mudra

Prithvi Mudra is formed by touching the frontal position of the thumb with the frontal portion of the ring finger. By practising this mudra tones down earth element is compensated and enhanced. It also enhances other elements in the body due to which body remains healthy and proper balance among all the elements remain well maintained. If body weight is less than the height of the body, this mudra restores proper proportion and balance between both the facets. Its practice also imparts lustre, glow and brightness to the face, and also inclines and motivates the mind towards spirituality. It also installs qualities of mercy, compassion and love, in addition to tolerance and patience.

Prana Mudra

Prana Mudra is formed by joining the front portion of little and ring finger with front portion of the thumb. This mudra acts like an electric stick because when this switch is pressed whole body gets infused with energy. Due to lack of Pranic energy, our body is embroiled with various ailments. One can always remain healthy and free from diseases by storing pranic energy in the body and this mudra helps a person fully to achieve his object of staying healthy. In reality, this mudra actually imparts 'Pran'. By continuous practice of this mudra, all eye-related diseases can be dispelled.

Apaan Mudra

Deficiency of inadequacy of Pran Vaayu is a causative factor for onset of many diseases. Impure and toxic matters can not be expelled from the body, if this element is found wanting, as a result of which impurities and diseases overpower human body. Hence our body can stay clear from such diseases and impurities if our body continues t o utilise Apaan Vaayu thus keeping balance within all the elements. Its use is like baking the body in fire so that blood is purified and body and mind are also purified of harmful substances. If any patient is suffering from urinary obstruction, due to any reason, he will pass urine within 15-20 minutes after practising this mudra. But, patients suffering from prostate gland and stone problems will not benefit from this Mudra. To restore the urinary flow, this mudra must be performed with both the hands.

If the pregnant ladies practise this mudra in the 8th month of pregnancy for 45 minutes daily, they will have an easy delivery and delivery will so take place at the expected time. If any pregnant lady finds it difficult to expel the baby or if delivery is getting delayed, she also can have an easy and natural delivery, provided she regularly practises this mudra.

If a person has suffered a heart attack, he should form this mudra with his left hand and also firmly compresses his right hand's thumb, middle and ring fingers himself or asks some another person to do the job for him, he will have an instant relief. This experiment has been used on many patients of heart attack and at all the occasions we were successful.

If a person has vomiting and loose motions (diarrhoea), he must not practise this mudra as he is most likely to be harmed.

Method- Bend the forefinger to touch the base of the thumb and join the tips of middle finger and ring finger with the tip of thumb.

Benefits - This mudra has proved to be the most wonderful treatment for coronary ailments. In emergency cases (like heart attack), this mudra shows its immediate effect on the heart patients like the sorbitrate tablet and patient gets miraculous relief in the form of first aid. That is why it is also called 'Mirtsanjivani Mudra'. If this mudra is practised regularly for a short period of time, then heart will slowly become quite strong. It also normalizes the pulse rate of the person.

Vyan Mudra

Method - Join the tip of forefinger and middle finger to the tip of thumb.

Benefits - This mudra if practised continuously to reduce the high blood pressure.

❑❑❑❑

10.
SHAT KARM
– THE CLEANSING EXERCISES

These yogic kriyas are the purification processes of the body by yogic methods. They are very important in Yoga. Union of body with mind, union of mind with soul and union of soul with God is Yoga.

Kriyas are to be practised early in the morning before rise on empty stomach. Kriyas must be finished before starting the Asanas or Pranayama.

These Kriyas consist of six purification practises –

1. Dhauti (Kunjal)
2. Basti
3. Neti
4. Tratak
5. Nauli, and
6. Kapalbhati.

Dhauti (Kunjal)

Vomit-Dhauti-Cleaning. Washing stomach by water.

Two or three litres of tepid water is required. Squat on your feet and your back, spine and neck should be straight. Drink glasses of tepid water continuously without any pause upto the brim of neck. One should neither talk nor laugh during this period. He should not bend and should stand.

Bend a bit forward. Keep the left hand on the left knee and the first and second finger of the right hand in your throat. Press the stomach by the other hand. You will vomit. Vomit the whole drunk water. Water should not remain in stomach.

Wash you hands and take rest. Milk or breakfast should be taken after an hour.

This Dhauti kriya should be practised after passing stool and after bath. One should not take bath after this kriya. Vaman Dhauti kriya should be practised once a fortnight or once a month.

Precautions -

- Heart patients should not practise it.
- The nails of the fingers should be trimmed otherwise they may wound the throat.

Benefits -

- Disorders of bile and gas are cured.
- It is beneficial in the diseases of stomach, throat and jaundice.

Basti (Enema)

Enema pot, rubber tube, nozzle, tepid water, lemon are the requirements. Mix juice of one or two lemons in the tepid water. Fill the enema pot with water.

Suspend the enema pot one metre above. Apply a little oil or vaseline to the nozzle of the rectal tube. Before insertion, check the rectal tube to ensure free flow of water. Insert the tube into the rectum. The flow of water can be adjusted with the knob attached to the tube. When all the water has been introduced, remove the tube and resist the pressure for a few minutes. The bowels can be emptied after a while for better cleansing. If one does not wish to take enema in the lying position he can take it in the standing position.

Note - Enema should be taken after going to latrine. Salt can be mixed in water instead of lemon juice. You can use plain water also. Soap should not be mixed in water.

Precautions -

- Enema should be taken once in a week or in a month by a healthy person.
- It can be taken for two to four days daily in constipation.
- Take rest for half an hour after enema.
- Do not take any thing after enema for an hour.

Benefits -

- Removes constipation.
- Cleans bowels.
- Beneficial in all diseases of stomach.

Neti

It is mainly of two types :

(i) Jala Neti (ii) Sutra Neti.

Jala Neti

For doing this, squat on your feet. Take tepid salted water in a medium sized pot with a long spout, made especially for this purpose.

Now fill the pot with tepid salted water and hold it in your right hand to the level of your nose. Then tilt your head slightly to the left so as to have the slanting position of the left nostril. Insert the nozzle of the spout into the right nostril and allow the water to flow down slowly. The water should continue falling down from other nostril in a continuous thin stream. Now repeat the process from the other side. Breath through the mouth only till the kriya is complete. After Jal Neti, stand erect with your feet together. Keep the hands behind your back clasped and blow out vigorously whatever trace of water that has remained in your nostrils.

Precautions - If sometimes one feels intolerable pain in the back of ear or above nostrils, he should practise the Kriya of Kapalbahit at once. It will cure the pain.

Water can come out of eyes in beginning of Neti. These can be warmed. Do not fear.

Benefits -

- It cures sinusitis and clears sinuses.
- It cures diseases of nose, eyes, throat and prevents the occurrence of diseases.
- It purifies mind.
- It improves memory.
- It cures coryza and removes old accumulated phlegm.

Sutra Neti or Rubber Neti

Sutra Neti is performed with a 12 inches long piece of waxed cord. It is partly twisted and it makes the nasal insertion possible.

Squat on your feet. Take tepid salted water and soak the Neti well in it. Now take the waxed and twisted end of the cord and make it to curve. Bend your head slightly forward and insert the end of the cord into the nostril through which you have been breathing at that time. Push the cord gradually through the nose, down the throat. Now open your mouth wide, put your index and middle fingers in and with their tips catch the inside end of the cord and draw it out. Hold both the ends in your hand separately and pull the cord very gently up and down three to four times. Then take it out, wash it and then repeat the cycle with the other nostril.

After completion of the kriya, wash the cord with soap well and leave it to dry in some clean and safe place so that the flies, etc. do not pollute it.

Special note -

- When the cord reaches throat through nostrils, it becomes greasy by mucurs. Therefore, both the ends of the cord should be caught firmly.
- Sutra Neti or Rubber Neti should be practised after learning Jal Neti. After this one can practise Neti with milk, oil or ghee.
- It is more beneficial to perform this Sutra Neti by cotton cord but it should be wrapped.

Precautions -

- One can sneeze in practising Sutra Neti. Water can come out of eyes. One should not fear. Practise makes one perfect.
- Nose can bleed sometimes while performing Sutra Neti. In such conditions use rubber catheter (No. 4) instead of cotton cord. Move the cord through nostrils and throat slowly and gently.

Benefits -

- It cures all diseases of nose.
- It reduces polyp in nose.
- It cures sinusitis.
- It cures coryza.
- It improves eyesight.
- It improves memory.
- It purifies mind.

Nasapan

Drinking water through nostrils is called nasapan. One should clean the nostrils before drinking water through them.

Milk Neti

Milk is used in place of water. Milk should be without malai (cream).

Benefits - Nasapan prevents cold and coryza. It improves eyesight.

Oil Neti

Mustard oil should be made warm in a spoon. When it is lukewarm and tolerable to the skin, lie down on a bed and drip five or seven drops of oil through some dropper in both the nostrils and try to draw them in. You will feel that the oil is going in. You can use clean cotton instead of dropper. Coconut or almond oil can be used in place of mustard of. Pure ghee can also be used. Three or four drops of ghee or badaam rogan are sufficient for the nostrils.

Oil Neti or Neti of ghee should be done before going to bed at night.

Benefits - It lubricates nose and cleanses it. It prevents from cold and coryza.

Tratak

It is an amazing exercise to improve your power of concentration and eyesight.

It can be practised with a candle or with a black dot on a piece of paper fixed on the wall. Start this practice in a closed room, as there will be less objects to disturb your concentration.

Sit on floor in any comfortable of Padmasana pose. Keep your back and spinal cord erect. Have a few deep breaths. Make your breath steady, even and rhythmic. Keep the object of your gaze at your eye level at a distance of three to four feet. Keep the eyes meditatively wide out of your eyes. Close the eyes to let tears trickle down.

Now mentally visualize that object when the mental image visualizes, open your eyes and start gazing afresh. Do not strain your nerves and get relaxed. Let not your mind wander. Try to bring your mind back to the object but without straining yourself much as that would sap your energy and you will be tired soon.

After practising with the point on the walls or on a steady flame, try to-do it concentrating on the tip of your nose on the point between the eyebrows.

Benefits -

- Tratak improves eyesight and removes the diseases of eyes.
- It helps in concentrating your mind.
- It purifies your mind.

Nauli Kriya

It is the best exercise for preserving and promoting the health of abdominal viscera.

- Nauli is equal to Uddiyana Bandh.
- Nauli should be practised daily in the morning on empty stomach and evacuated bowels.
- Stand with legs one foot apart. Bend the legs a little and stoop forward. Rest the palms on thighs just above your knees, with fingers spread. Press the thighs well with your palms and the chest with your chin at the notch between the collar bones.
- Inhale deeply and exhale vigorously so as to force out all the air from the lungs.
- Suspend the breath and pull the abdominal region back towards the spine so that a hollow is formed.
- Push the abdominal recti forward so that a vertical ridge down the centre is formed. Remain in this position for a few seconds and then relax the gap and inhale smoothly.
- Breath deeply three to four times and then repeat the cycle. Repeat it five to seven times.

Special note -

1. Nauli kriya is not easy. Obese persons feel difficulty in its practise. It is essential to practice Uddiyana Bandh and Agnisar to perform Nauli.

2. Nauli kriya should be performed on empty stomach after cleaning bowels and before taking food.
3. One should wear only underwear while practising Nauli. Women can wear bra/ brassiere also.

Precautions-

- Nauli should be practised on empty stomach.
- It should not be practised unless there is some expert to demonstrate and then to guide and supervise the whole process.
- It should not be practised before the age of 12 or 13 years.
- The ulcer patient and the weak person should perform Nauli on the advice of Yoga therapist.
- The patients suffering from swelling of intestines, dysentery, hernia and high blood pressure should not practice Nauli.

Benefits - The benefits of Nauli are many. It strengthens the abdominal muscles and liver. Women who suffer from a menstrual problem get immediate relief. It increases gastric fire and helps eliminating the toxic elements from the digestive system. It also helps in ovarian insufficiency. Nauli quickly cures constipation, dyspepsia, flatulence etc.

Kapalbhati

Kapal means skull. Bhati means shine or lustre. Thus, this term means "skull shining". Kapalbhati is a Pranayama also besides one of the six cleaning exercises. Actually this kriya or cleansing process is a milder form of Bhastrika, another vigorously breathing exerci se.

Sit on a blanket or a dari in Padmasana, Sidhasana or Sukhasana. Keep back, spinal cord and neck erect. Keep both the hands on knees. Shut your eyes. Sit peacefully. Exhale vigorously. Do not inhale. At start begin slowly after four to five exhales exhale vigorously and quickly. Be careful in exhaling; you will inhale between exhales.

One should not pause during the practice of Kapabhati. Hold the breath after exhaling (Kumbhak). During Kumbhak practice Jallandhar Bandh, Uddiyana Bandh, Mool Bandh and Mahabandh. Hold this position for a while. Release all Bandhs and inhale slowly. This completes one round of Kapalbhati. Start with two rounds. You can practice unto five rounds gradually. Start with ten or twelve exhales. Gradually you can increase their number 50 to 120.

Special Note -

1. The stomach should go inside at once after exhaling.
2. The difference between Kapabhati and Bhastrika Pranayma is that both inhale and exhale are done vigorously. One should learn it from an expert in Yogic Kriya.

Precautions - Persons with high blood pressure or pus in the ear should refrain from doing this exercise.

Benefits - This Kapalbhati is very good invigorating exercise which cleanses the entire respiratory system by forcefully rushing exhalation.

It removes concentration and mental retention. The movement of the diaphragm stimulates the stomach, heart liver and spleen. This exercise is very good for eyes.

Agnisar

The practice of Agnisar kindles energy in stomach and body perspires.

Sit on a blanket or dari in Vajrasana. Keep a little distance between the knees. Put firmly both the hands on the knees. Inhale vigorously and while exhaling shrink your stomach as much as you can. Now suspend your breath. It is called Bahya Kumbhak.

Holding the position of Bahya Kumbhak, i.e. keeping the breath suspended and pulling the entire abdominal region back towards your spine. Now blow your stomach out and shrink in. In one Kumbhak you can blow and shrink your stomach 8-20 times.

This kriya is called Agnisar. One can practice this kriya in a standing posture.

Benefits -

- Cures obesity.
- Cures disorders of abdominal region.
- It improves lack of appetite.

11.
SURYA NAMASKAR – EK CHAMATKAR

Sun is supposed to be the best source of energy. The Asana by which Sun is worshipped is called 'Surya namaskar'. This consists of 12 steps and with every step, Sun is worshipped by a specific Mantra.

This asana is supposed to be complete in itself. Anybody, of any sex, at any age, can perform this asana . This should be done smoothly and slowly. No other asana should be performed before or after Surya Namaskar. Neither jogging nor brisk walking is required before or after Surya Namaskar. This asana should be performed by keeping face towards Sun in early morning.

Caution - Patients/persons suffering from heart problems, having high/low blood pressure or during fever, this asana should not be performed.

First Step - Stand on a blanket or mat keeping your face in front of the Sun. Join the knees, heels and feet of both legs. Keep your back, spinal cord and head in a straight position. Join both the hands and bend the elbow in a position of Namaskar. This is first step. Now repeat silently - *'OM Mitroya Namah'*. (Friend Sun, I salute you).

Second Step - Raise both your arms by inhaling. Stop breathing. Keeping air inside your lungs. Bend your back, neck, head and arms backwards. Legs should not bend and keep your body in this position for some seconds. This is second step. Repeat - *(OM Ravya Namah).* (May Sun! you are capable of keeping this world mobile so I salute you)

Third Step - Now release your holded breath and bend yourself forward. Touch your both palms to earth and your forēhead should touch the knees. There should be no bend in knees as shown in fig. 3. This is third step. Repeat-*'OM Suryay Namah'* (Sun, you are capable of providing life to this world, so I salute you).

Fourth Step - The palms should be touched to earth and start inhaling, as shown in fig. 4. Raise your left leg backwards. Bend your right knee and keep it on sole. Keep your chest ahead. Bend your neck backwards. Look forward to the sky. This is fourth step. Recall Sun in your mind with the Mantra - *'OM Bhanve Namah'* (Hey! source of light, I salute you).

Fifth Step - Straight your both arms, keeping your palms on the earth. Start taking breath and raise your right leg too backwards as shown in fig. 5. Now keep both the legs parallel. But there should be no gap in between heels and knees of both legs. The whole weight of the body should be on palms and soles. Now repeat in mind - *'OM Khagaya Namah'* (Hey! Sun you are able for motion in sky, I salute you).

Sixth Step - Hold the breath in lungs and keeping your palms and soles on earth, bend your elbows and touch your chest and knees to earth. This is called 'Ashtaang Pranaam', as shown in fig. 6. In this position light organs of the body touch the earth i.e. two soles, two hands, chest, forehead and two knees; so why it is called 'Ashtaang Pranaam'. This is the sixth step. Now remember Sun by repeating in your mind - 'OM Pushney

Namah' - (Hey! Sun, you are providing food to world, I salute you).

Seventh Step - Keep your palms on earth and straight your arms, keeping breath. Raise your upper portion of the body upto naval pit. Keep ahead your chest and bend your neck backwards. Look forwards sky. Raise your legs backwards, keeping your soles towards sky. This is step seven as shown in fig. 7. Now repeat - *'OM Hiranya Garbhaya Namah'* - (As you are a light source, I salute you).

Eighth Step - Keep your palms on the earth. Exhale the breath and raise both the legs towards hands. Raise the hips straight. Keep soles, feet and palms in touch of earth. Keep your head in between of the arms. Raise your back as shown in fig. 8. There should be no gap in between both legs. Keep your stomach inside & hold the breath outside. Now remember Sun by repeating in mind - *'Om Marichaye Namah'* - (Sun, you are all in all, so I salute you).

Ninth step - Continue the retention of breath. Place hands and feet firmly on the ground. Lift your bottoms. Press your chin to the chest. Stomach should be drawn in.

Tenth Step - While sitting on the ground, put the left foot forward and right foot backward stretchingly. Try to touch your front foot with your fingers of hands. The throat should be between the two arms and erect. Stomach should be drawn in. Bring the right foot forward and draw the left foot backwards stretchingly. Try to touch the front foot with fingers of both hands. This improves blood circulation, stengthens the feet and makes the spinal cod elastic.

Eleventh step - Drawng the stomach in join both legs. Touch the kness with your nose. Exhale with nose. This strengthens fingers, hands, chest and stomach.

Twenth step - Inhale with nose. Stand erect and join feet and knes. Keep the hands folded and touching firmly your chest.

Advantages of Surya Namaskar

- By practising Surya Namaskar in winter, you will be free from cold, cough and coryza.
- Eye sight is improved.
- Shoulders are strenghened and abdominal diseases are cured.
- The mind becomes tension free and mind power is increased.
- The spinal cord becomes elastic and muscles are strengthened surrounding spinal cord.
- Blood circulation of whole body is accelerated and diseases of respiratory system are and diseases of respiratory system are annihilated.
- Ligaments are strengthened.
- Body becomes vigorous and glowing.

□□□□

Shatkarma – The Cleansing Exercise

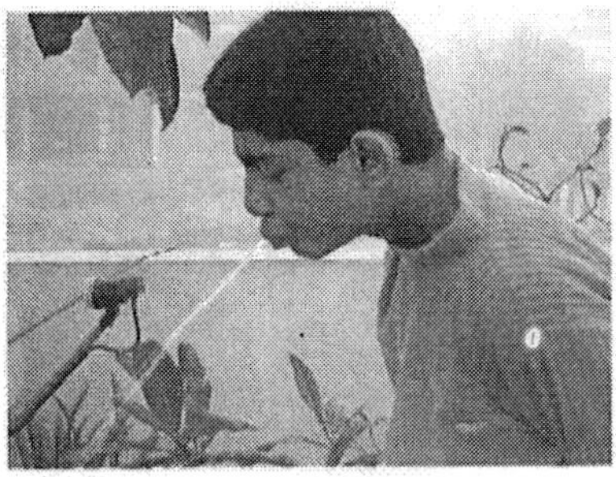

Dhauti

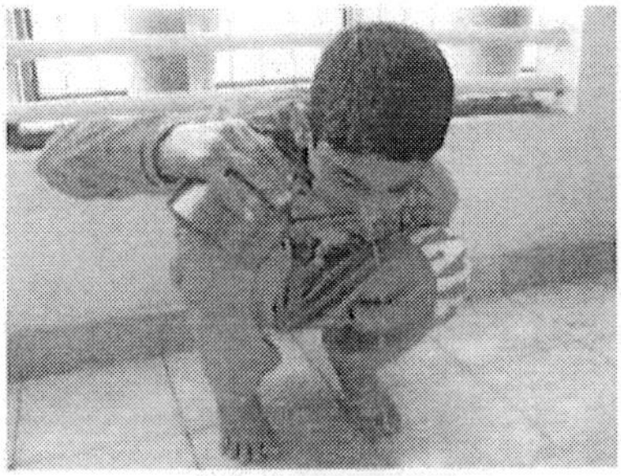

Jal Neti

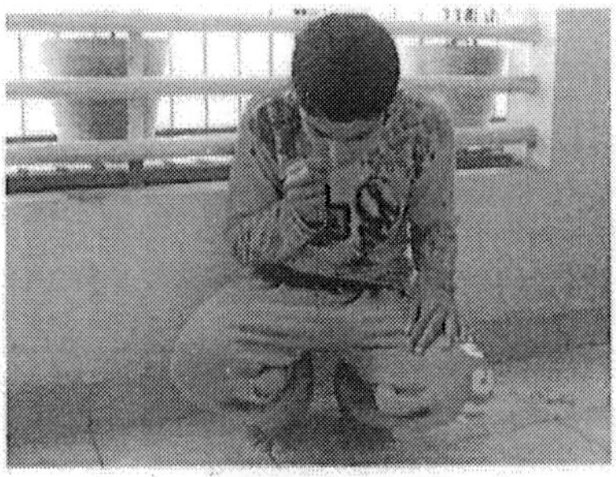

Sutra Neti

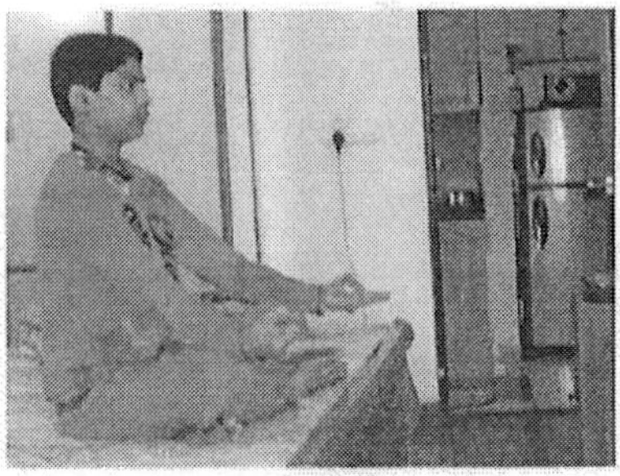

Tratak

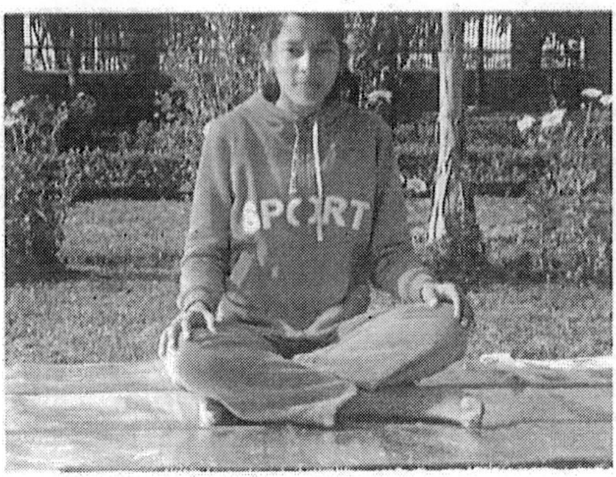

Kapalbhati

Surya Namaskar
Ek Chamatkar

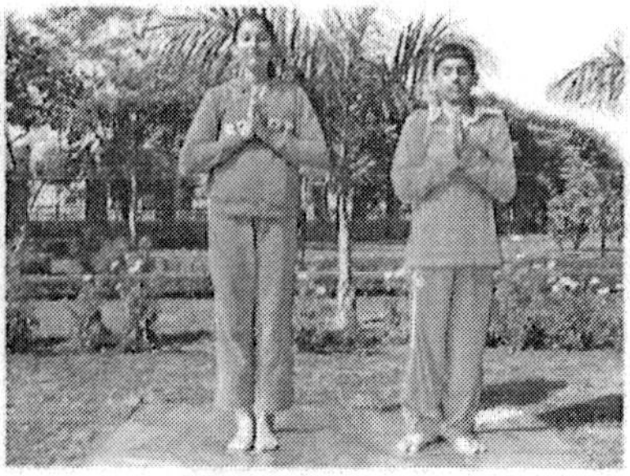

Surya Namaskar 1.

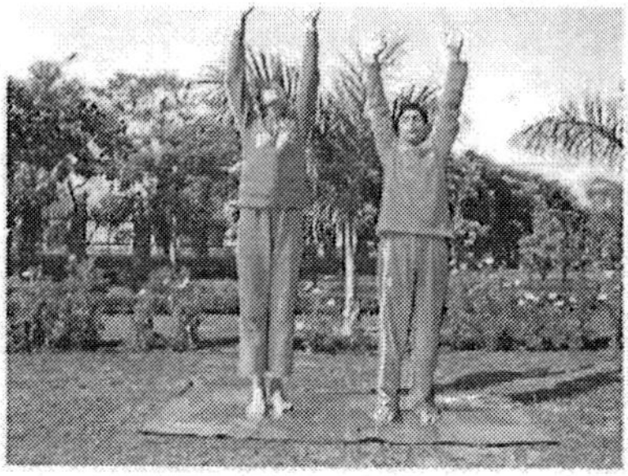

Surya Namaskar 2.

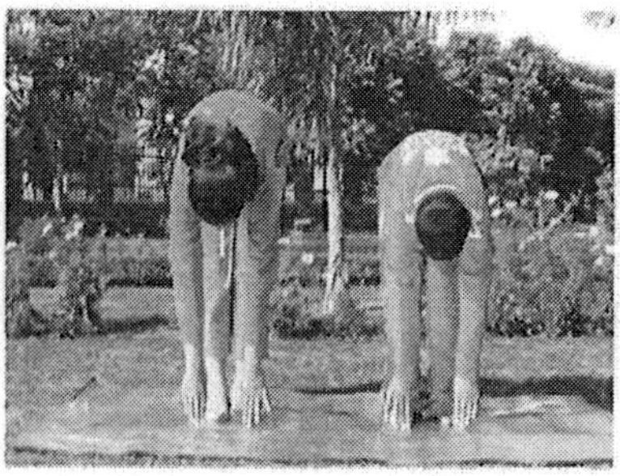

Surya Namaskar 3.

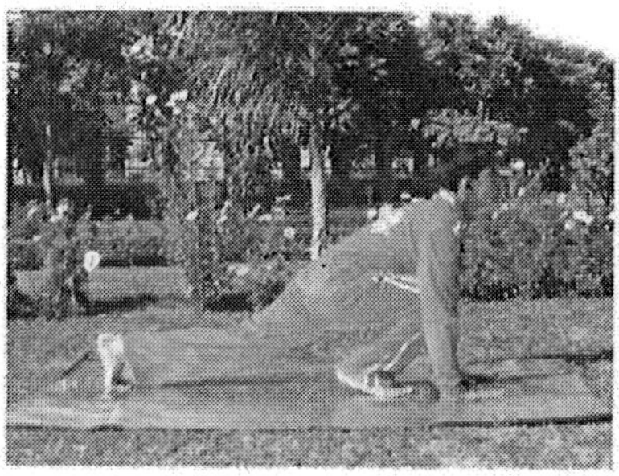

Surya Namaskar 4.

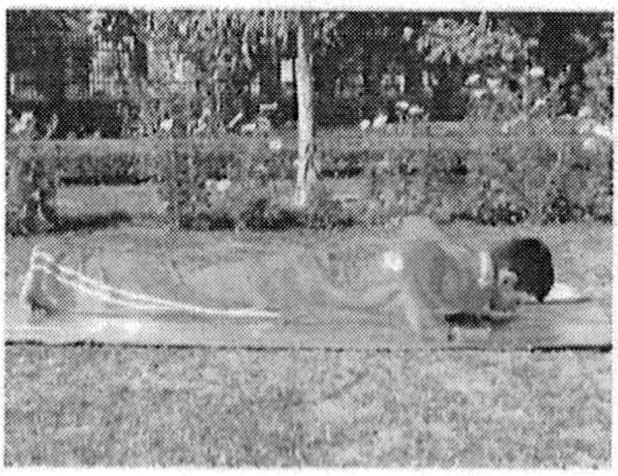

Surya Namaskar 5.

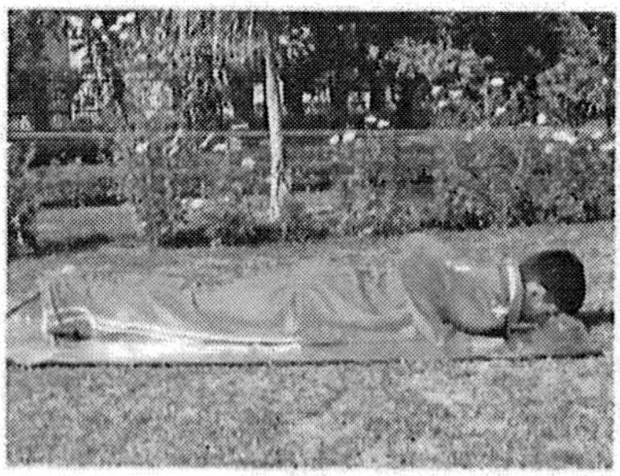

Surya Namaskar 6.

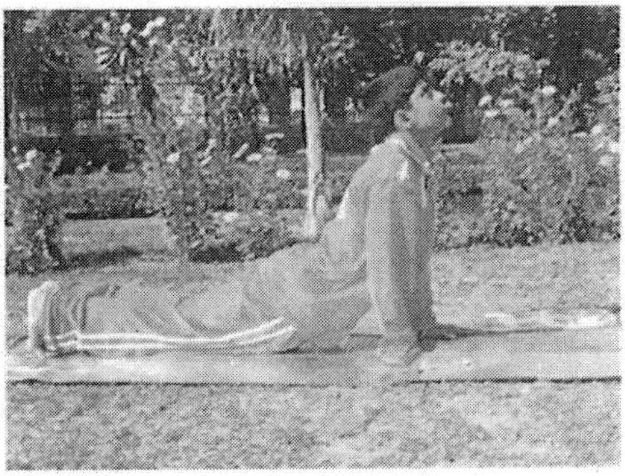

Surya Namaskar 7.

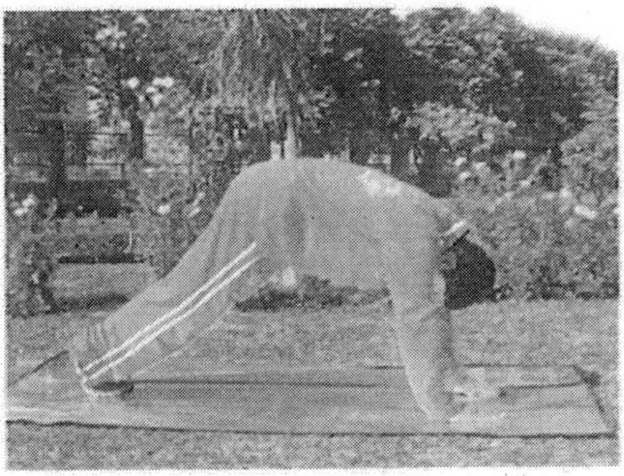

Surya Namaskar 8.

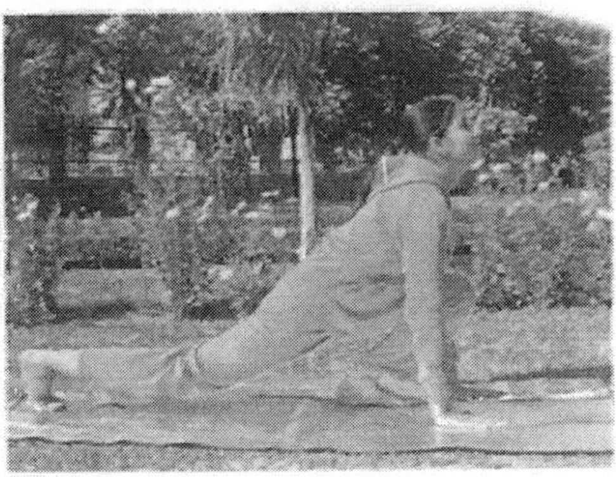

Surya Namaskar 9.

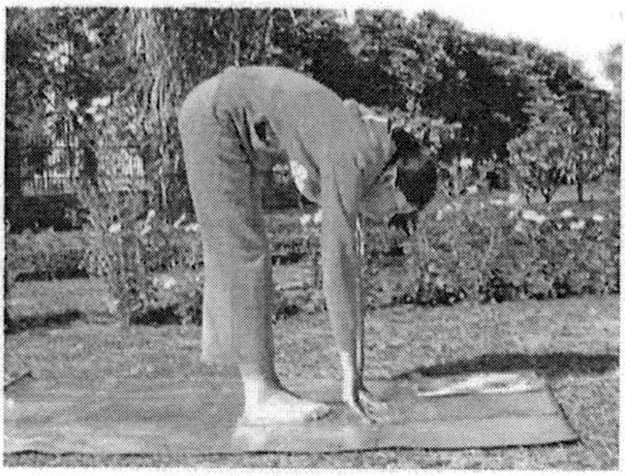

Surya Namaskar 10.

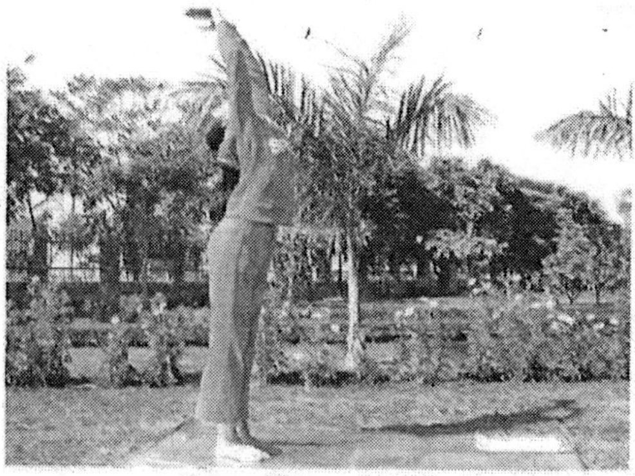

Surya Namaskar 11.

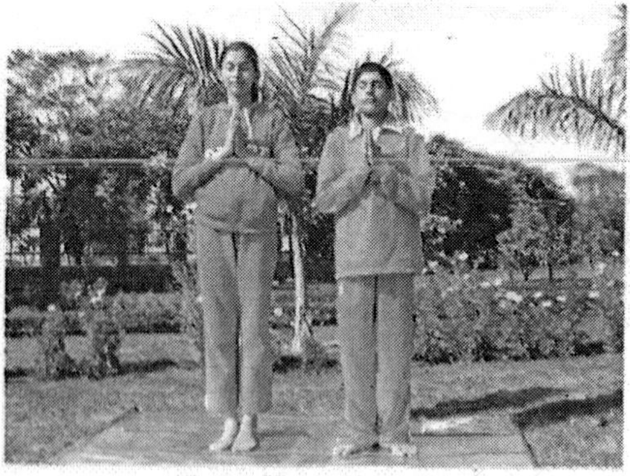

Surya Namaskar 12.

Powerful Yogic Exercises – Bandha (Locks)

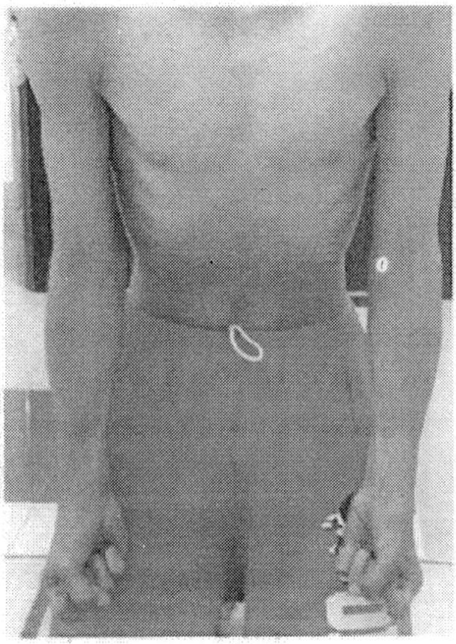

Nauli (Uddiyan Bandh)

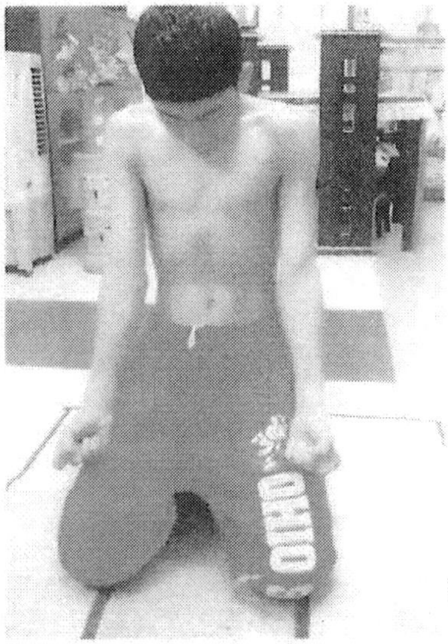

Two Bandhs
(Nouli & Jalandhar in one pose)

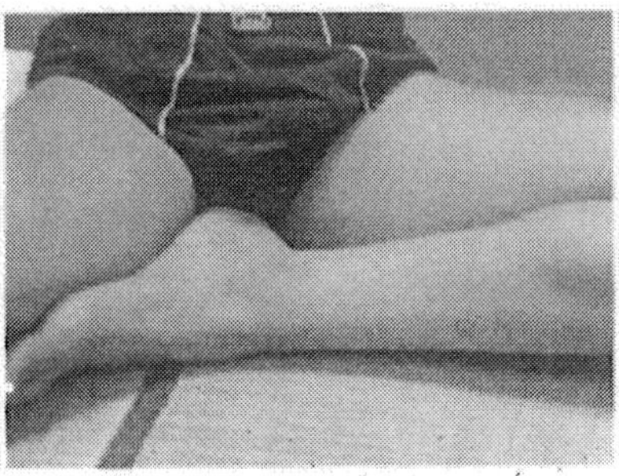

Moola Bandh

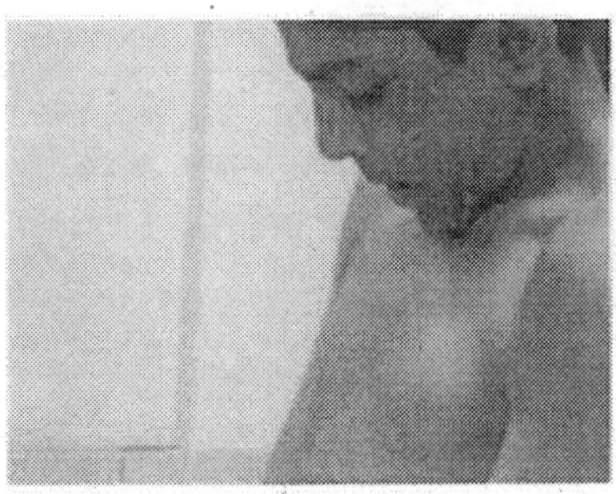

Jalandhar Bandh

Pranayama – It's Healing Powers and Benefits

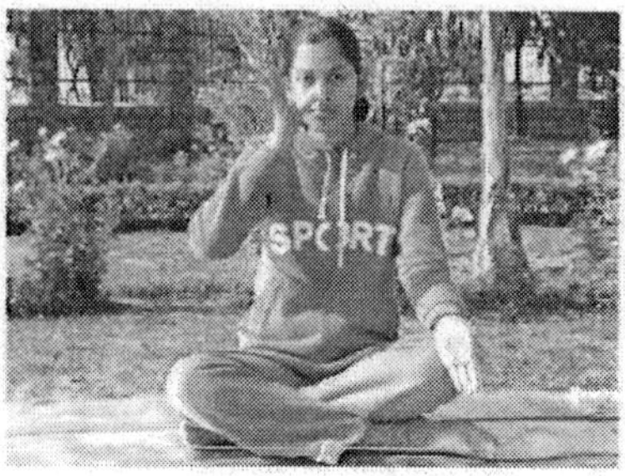

Pranayama 1. Inhale

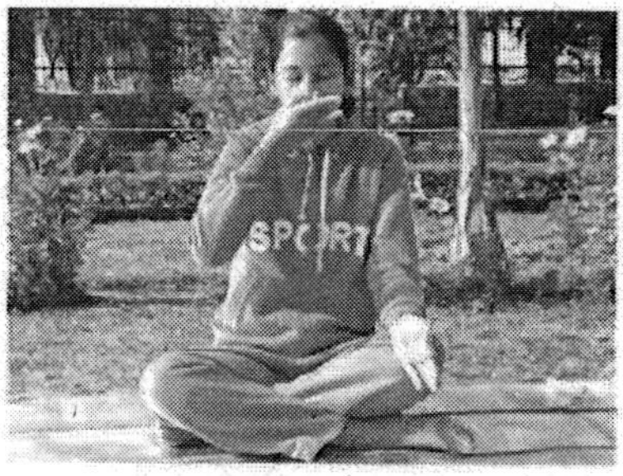

Pranayama 2.
Hold and then exhale from other nostril keeping close the opposite nostril

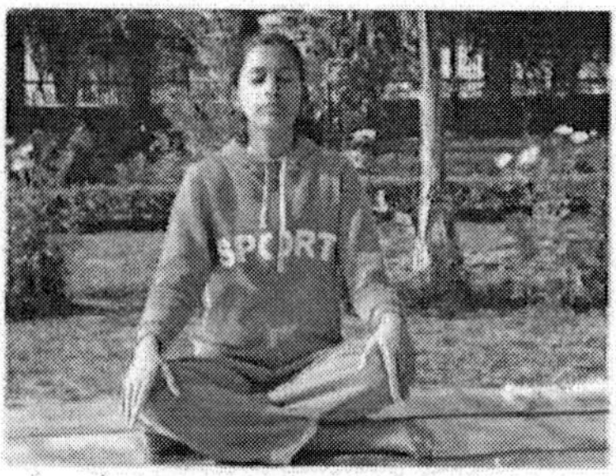

Deep breathing and then open the eyes after a short while slowly

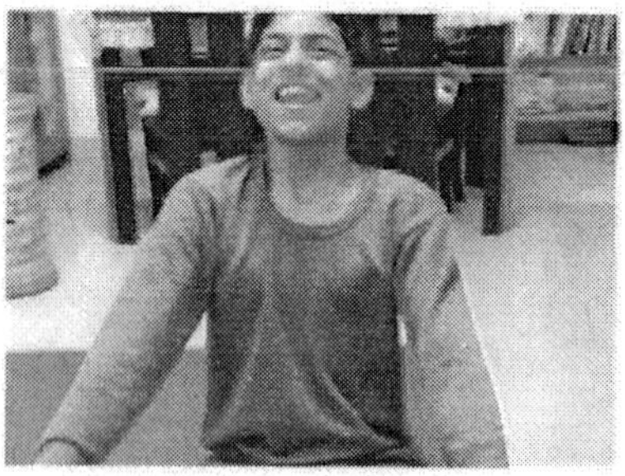

Shitali Pranayama

Meditation – The Scientific Way

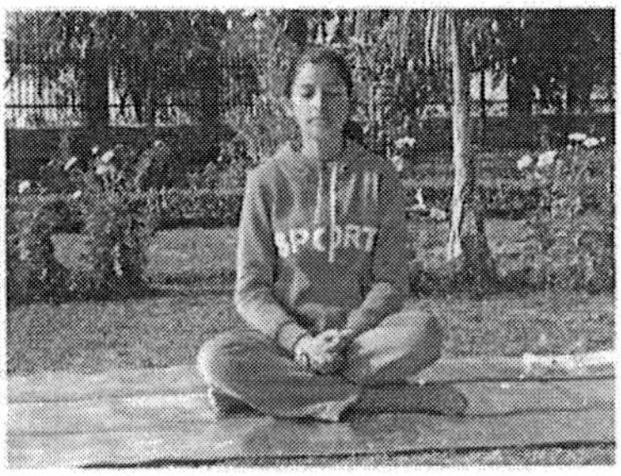

Meditattion 1.

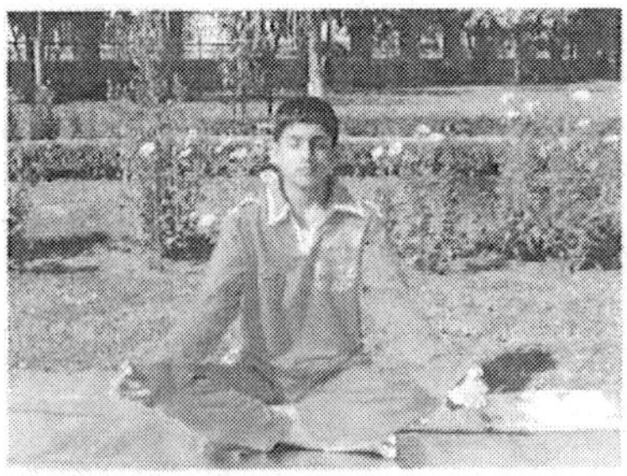

Meditattion 2.

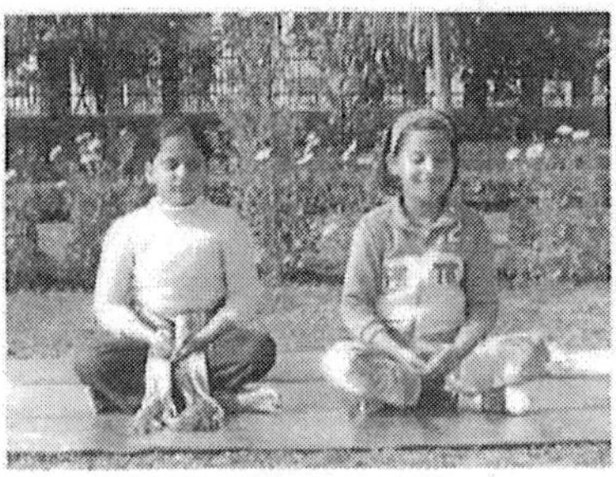

Meditattion 3.

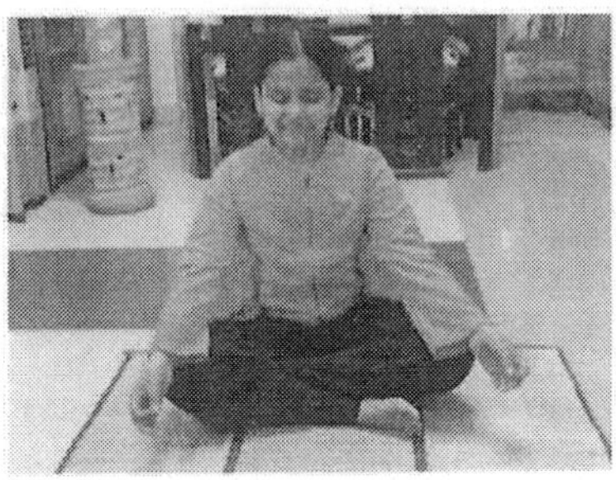

Meditate and feel pleasure inside
to relieve stress

Yogic Exercise for Relaxation

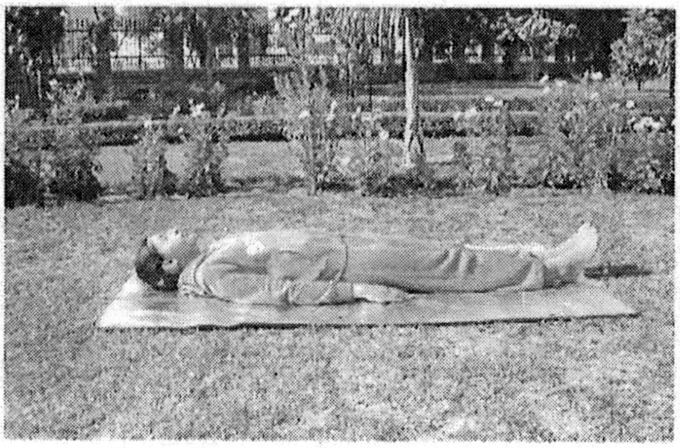

Shavsana 1.

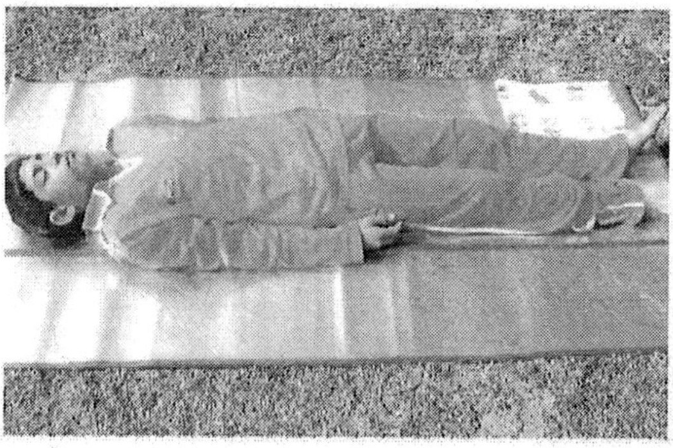

Shavsana 1.

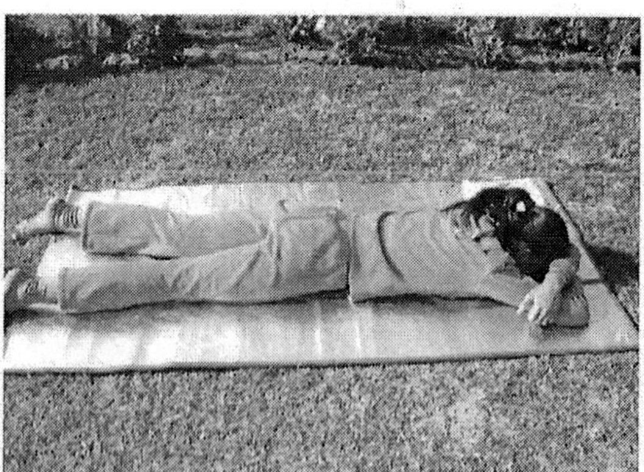

Makrasana

12.
POWERFUL YOGIC EXERCISES – BANDHA (LOCKS)

This is a very powerful and important practice of Yoga. It is very helpful in gaining perfect control over all the parts of the body and nerves. Bandha (lock) means to tie up or to make something stiff or to keep under control. It massages the internal organs. Although it is a physical practice that makes the functioning of body balanced and helps in attaining to better health, yet, at the same time, it also controls the thoughts and vibrations from the soul and has a subtle effect on the chakras. Thus, lock leads to spiritual progress and activation of the dormant powers in the body. In other words, lock helps in removing the obstruction in the sushumna channel and in promoting free flow of pranic energy through it. This leads to activation of several glands and helps one to have the highest experience of Yoga.

It is for this final accomplishment of liberation that asanas, pranayama, mudras and bandhas are practised. Hence, through perfect harmony between the Yogic processes, the spiritual energies are activated and spiritual powers are attained and one reaches one's final goal.

Bandha Locks Jalandhara Bandha (Water Gate Lock Or Chiin Lock)

Sit in padmasana or siddhasana or perform this practice while standing. Place your hands on the knees. Relax the entire body and close the eyes. Breathe in, deeply and, then, hold the breath in. Bend your head forward and press the chin into the chest. Straighten the hands and pressing the knees sit still or be in standing still. Position the shoulders a bit forward with both of them raised a bit. Keep the entire body, stiff and still. This is the position of jalandhara bandha. Hold the breath in, i.e., internal retention and try to remain in this position for as long as you can, comfortably. Then, relax the shoulders and hands and raise the head. Breathe out, slowly. Rest, for some time and, then, repeat.

One can also perform the Bandha in another way. Breathe in deeply, then, without holding in the breath, breathe out, completely. Then, perform the bandha holding the breath out, i.e., external retention. Concentrate on the vishuddhi chakra.

Precautions - Those suffering from high blood pressure, heart problems, mental stress and migraine should practice under the guidance of a Yoga expert.

Benefits - This practice affects the nerves of the neck, the arteries that carry blood to the head, the thyroid and parathyroid glands, etc. Thus, the shape and development of the body and the sexual performance get regulated. It also helps in getting rid from mental tension, worries, anger and mental disorders. It also helps control disorders related to high and low blood pressure.

Mula Bandha (Root Lock or The Anal Lock)

Sit in any meditative pose with the knees touching the floor. For this, siddhasana is best. In this lock, the muladhara region is contracted. Thus, mula bandha, i.e., the anal lock is performed, automatically. Close the eyes and place the palms on the knees. Relax the entire body. Breathe in deeply and hold the breath in, i.e., internal tension. Then, perform jalandhara bandha. Contract and relax the sphincter muscles and try to pull them, inwards. This is the final position. Try to hold the breath in for as long as you can and keep contracting and relaxing the sphincter muscles. Finally, relax the muscles and relax the lock. Then, slowly breathe out. Concentrate on the midadhara chakra.

One can also do this practice after exhaling, completely and holding the breath out, i.e., external retention. Those who wish to remain in the final position for a long time can do so by breathing, normally.

Benefits - In this practice, the apana vayu mixes with prana vayu, i.e., the excretory air merges into the life force called as vital air and this results in generation of a great amount of energy that helps in activation of kundalin more easily. This practice is helpful in maintenance of celibacy and activation of divine energy within. It is also very beneficial for those suffering from piles, indigestion and other stomach ailments. It tones up and strengthens the sphincter muscles, the nerves of the waist region and the intestines. It prepares the mind for spiritual practices.

Uddiyana Bandha (Abdominal Lock)

Sit in a meditative pose in which the knees touch the floor. Padmasana and Sidhasana are best. Place the palms on the knees. Breathe out, completely and holding the breath out, i.e., external retention perform jalandhara bandha. Now, pull the stomach inwards and upwards as much as you can, i.e., total contraction of abdomen. Remain in the final position comfortably. Type of worshipping can also be of three types - Vedic, smarta and laukika.

For Vedic worship, one has to, first, learn the proper pronunciation of the Vedic mantras and also know about the

(the seer of the mantra), chanda (the metre of the mantra), devata (deity), brija (the code of the mantra), gakti (the trigger), Maka (lock) and viniyoga (the offering) related to a particular mantra, the syllable. One has to daily have a bath before starting the practice. One has to wear fresh clothes, sit on a particular worship-mat with a pure heart and meditate on the divine form of the deity, after having performed rsyadi nyasa (establishing the etc., in our body in different specific organs who created that particular practice), (to establish the diety, etc., in the different parts of our body) and karanyasa (to establish the deity, etc., in the different fingers of our hand). These are very essential for the purification of all the parts of our body, before using a particular practice for prayer, without which the deity cannot be pleased. If there is a special verse for meditation, then, one should contemplate on the divine form of the deity in one's heart and devote oneself on his feet. Thereafter, one should chant the Vedic mantra 2, 3, 5, 11, 21, 51, 108'or, more times, with full concentration. In the end, one should offer one's chanting into the feet of the deity to appease

□□□□

13.
BREATHING PROCESS AND ELEMENTS OF PRANA

Prana is the sustaining force of human body. As long as prana exists in the body, life persists and, when prana leaves it, death ensues. Right from birth to death, prana is all-pervasive. It is the be-all and end-all of human existence. Prana is nurtured by five elements, Viz.

1. Air
2. Water
3. Earth
4. Akash and
5. Fire

The above mentioned five elements, when in balanced and equilibrium, help the human body to sustain itself but, when this balance is disturbed, a diseased state sets in. Disease is nothing but simply state of a disordered air which is the most predominant factor, as we cannot live or breathe in and breathe out without air, though we can live without the rest of four elements for sometime. Next to air comes water and then the remaining elements.

Human body is composed of two parts viz.

(i) The visible physical body and

(ii) The invisible energy body (also called 'The Bioplasmic Energy'.)

Visible physical body is that which we touch, see and hear. Bioplasmic body is an invisible luminous energy body that inter penetrates the visible physical body and extends beyond it by 4 to 5 inches and clairvoyants prefer to call the "energy body", "the etheric body" or "etheric double."

Whenever a person is infected by some ailment, his ailing organ/part indicates lack or inadequate energy flow. When the life energy or Ki is replenished, a state of health returns. As long as life energy permeates to each organ and sinew of body, there is hardly any chance of facing any health hazard. The heater transmits life energy to his patient through various means, like psychic healing, therapeutic healing, vitalic healing, magnetic healing, faith healing, charismatic healing. In some cases, some saints and holy men simply rid the patient of his illness by looking deep into his eyes (which, in fact, is kind of establishment of visual contact between the patient and the healer). In short, a healer projects Prana to the patient.

I would compare Pranic energy to air filling in a tube. If too much air volume is created, the filled in tube can burst and, if too less of air is filled, there are chances the same may get damaged and cracked. There must be reasonable vacuum in a tube so that there is sufficient scope for the air to revolve therein. Let us compare this analogy to human body. When body is overloaded with too much eatables, it gets bloated but, when it is sparsely fed, it creates near starvation position hence, to keep the body in good humour, feed your body only with requisite diet. It is well said, "We are what we eat, that is to say that food choices (or better say 'food preferences') govern our habits and inclinations. If physical body is continuously starved of requisite nutritional diet, it is bound to adversely affect various functions of our body.

Following aspects greatly impact our Pranic efficiency.

1. Process of breathing
2. Five Koshas (or Five sheaths)
3. Chakras
4. Endocrine Glands
5. Nadis--the pathways of Pranic Current
6. Power of Mantras
7. Meridians
8. Disease
9. Food
10. Environmental effects
11. Psychic disorders

Lower end of trachea divides into smaller tubes called left and right bronchi, which further divide into smaller bronchioles (like the branches of an upside-down tree). The large bronchi retain small and smooth muscles and cartilage that prevent them from closing. As soon as these bronchial tubes become smaller, the cartilage disappears, and only a celiated mucus lining and fibrous muscular coat are left behind. The bronchioles terminate at small dilated air-tubes (called 'Alveoli') which are lined by capillaries and exchange of oxygen and carbon dioxide takes place between air and blood.

The lungs

The inner structure of lungs resembles a tree whose main trunk is trachea, bronchi and bronchioles the branches and leaves being the alveoli. There is a lung each on left and right sides of the chest, and lung tissue is pink and coloured (when in an unpolluted state) due to presence of blood capillaries. The left lung has only two lobes/compartments (while the right lung has three lobes) due to the fact that heart occupies room in the left ribcage. Each lung is elastic, spongy and porous, due to the presence of air in its alveoli, as if it floats on water.

The lungs are caged in a ribcage (thorax) and are separated, from the stomach and other digestive organs, by the diaphragm which lies where the ribs terminate or end. Pleura (double membrane) surrounds the lungs and provides a lubricating surface, between the inner chest cavity and the lungs, during the motions or movements of breathing. Heart sends impure blood to the lungs for oxygenation and expulsion of carbon dioxide. After purifying process, the lungs send back purifies and oxygenated blood to the heart to enable it to feed the physical system.

The Rib-cage

This is also called a thoracic cavity, within which heart is contained. The ribcage comprises of bones, muscles and cartilege and helps the air to pump in and pump out. The lungs are passive but have the capacity to inflate and deflate due to the impact of movement of the walls and floor of the throracic cavity. The thorax is bound by 12 thoracic vertebrae of the spine. The sternum or the breastbone lies in front of the 12 pairs of ribs that encircle the heart and lungs from the vertebral column at the back. The thoracic ribcage protects the vital organs from damage. The spaces between the ribcage contain inter costal muscles that connect them and also impart movement capacity to the ribcage. The ribs are articulated at each end so that they can move outwards and upwards.

The Diaphragm

Diaphragm performs major part of respiration, as ribcage can produce only a limited range of contraction and expansion of lungs. Diaphragm is a dome-shaped organ which has sheet of muscles and tendons attached to the lower ribs, and bulging upwardly into the thoracic cavity. It also forms a dividing partition between thoracic and abdominal cavities. It is an important organ from where oesophagus, vagus nerve and main vein (vena cava) and artery (aorta) to and for the lower body, pass through openings in the diaphragm.

On inhalation the diaphragm expands and raises upwardly while, on exhalation, it contracts. During inhalation the abdomen should bloat and expand but contract and squeeze when air is expelled. However, muscular effort is required, in both cases of inhalation and exhalation. Peristaltic action of the diaphragm massages and stimulates abdominal viscera, helps in digestion, assimilation and excretion.

Breath Volumes (including lung volume)

When we breathe in air, during the course of inhalation, but ded breathing, when we inhale about half a litre air, even though full capacity of lungs works to 4 ½ - 5 litres the former is called 'Tidal Volume, and the latter is called 'Vital capacity'. Inhalation and exhalation can be increased/decreased up-and-down the tidal volume. Despite all this, some volume of air always remain in the lungs, even if we feel that entire air volume has been exhaled. This is called 'Residual Volume'which is slightly more than one litre.

When atmospheric air is inhaled, we inhale

- 0.04% carbon dioxide (which is poison).
- 20% oxygen (which is body's life force).
- 79% Nitrogen (which doesn't play any role in our respiratory process).

But when air is exhaled following changes are generally noticed, that is

- There is no change in percentage of Nitrogen
- Carbon dioxide increases to around 4.04%. Oxygen is reduced to 16%.

It may be noted that cold air as inhaled and more humid and warm air is exhaled, due to water vapour exhalation from the lungs. During exhalation 1/5th of our body's heat is lost.

Respiration

The term 'Respiration' implies both the processes of inhalation and exhalation. Breathing is a natural phenomenon and pace of breathing varies from one person to another. Normally an adult breathes 15 breaths per minute which number can increase or decrease in view of one's physical, emotional and mental states as also due to environmental influences. Nervous and chemical controls are the two factors that control and regulate air respiratory mechanism.

Breathing is a natural, silent and uninterrupted process. When breathing process is in order everything else is in perfect order but, when breathing process is disturbed, nothing else can be in order, as a body without breath is a dead entity. If, we, have to survive, we have to breathe so that oxygen is supplied to the body to let it function normally. The marvel of breathing lies in continuous and unemployed breathing, as we continue to breathe, even if we are asleep or awake. When we are asleep, the subconscious mind supervenes but, during activity or awakened state conscious mind takes control of our body. This fact will be laid open and discussed, in greater details, when dealing with 'Pranayama'.

Nose and its Utility

Imagine what would be the condition of any person when both the nostrils get blocked, due to accumulation of thick, tenacious and sticky mucus, and one is obliged to breathe through mouth. When one has to breathe through mouth, tongue and throat membranes get dried up. Moreover, mouth breathing is only an emergent device and can never replace nasal breathing. Further, during mouth breathing all the foreign matters gain entry into our body.

Nose is the only organ that imparts us sense of smell and also helps to build up taste and liking for food. Nose has a direct connection with our brain, and its nostrils are the doorways that affect our entire mental and physical systems. Respiration gets impeded, if nostrils are blocked or choked. In order to facilitate breathing, without any hassles, try to keep your nasal passages clear by Pranayama, deep breathing, 'Neti Kriya', or steam inhalation. If nasal passages get frequently blocked yard respiration becomes a problem, seek help of a yoga expert.

If you have a blocked nose, you are most likely to develop catarrhal headache which may even percolate to eyes, temples, neck, check bones, sinuses. If there are hard crusts in the nose do not remove them forcibly, as you are likely to cause nasal bleeding and resultant wounds. Constant discharge or flow or obstruction may even damage septum and cartilages. Clear your nasal passages with saline water (cold or lukewarm). For free respiration, nasal passages must be free from all types of obstructions, including polypi, crusts, thick and tenacious mucus which is difficult to detach.

The Respiratory System

The Respiratory System enables oxygen from the air to be taken into the bloodstream to provide the energy to the body to meets its needs to function. As we breathe in, air is filtered by the nose, then travels via the windpipe (trachea) and bronchial tubes to the lungs, into millions of tiny sacs. Oxygen passes through the thin sac walls into the blood, in exchange for carbon dioxide, a waste product, which is breathed out. Mucus may collect in little-used parts of the lungs, encouraging bacteria to grow. In urban areas the air is often laden with chemicals from industry and traffic, placing a strain on the respiratory mucous membranes' defences.

Treatment aims to reduce the intake of pollutants and allergens, and lessen their effects on the lungs. Building up the immune system helps the body resist attack by micro-organisms inhaled through the nose and mouth.

Infections of the respiratory tract are often triggered by viruses. Irritation of the mucous membranes may constrict the airways, making breathing difficult. Decongestants, antihistamines and bronchodilators may be prescribed. Any secondary bacterial infections (those which occur after viral infections) are treated using antibiotics.

Air inhaled via the nose or mouth enters the windpipe (trachea) in the throat. The trachea divides into two tubes (bronchi) which enter the lungs–spongy, elastic air-filled organs to either side of the heart. Within each lung, the bronchi branch into smaller and smaller and tubes. The very smallest tubes (bronchioles) carry air into tiny sacs (alveoli) which are surrounded by microscopically fine blood vessels (capillaries), whose walls are so thin that oxygen from the air easily diffuses through them and into the red blood corpuscles, where it is carried in haemoglobin to body tissues. The respiratory tract is lined with mucous membranes.

The Theory of Relaxation & Breathing

With each breath, oxygen is absorbed into the blood, enabling production of the energy that fuels every body function. Under stress, breathing tends to be rapid, using the top half of the lungs. This causes a drop in blood levels of carbon dioxide, whiter is needed to maintain blood acidity. This can lead to tiredness and anxiety and create tension in the upper back, shoulders and neck. Abdominal breathing, which allows the lungs to expand full is a more efficient and calm way to breathe, and has the potential to benefit both physical and mental health.

Abdominal Breathing

Abdominal, or diaphragmatic, breathing uses the diaphragm the sheet of muscle that forms the floor of the chest cavity and the ceiling of the abdomen. On breathing in, the diaphragm contracts and moves downward rather like the piston of a bicycle pump. At the same time, the abdomen rises and the chest expands slightly as air is drawn in. On breathing out, the diaphragm relaxes and rises, making the space inside the chest cavity smaller and expelling air from the lungs.

How Oxygen Reaches the Bloodstream

As air is drawn into the lungs, alveoli (air sacs) transfer oxygen into the bloodstream and remove carbon dioxide from it.

Physiological Effects of Stress & Relaxation

Stressful situations trigger the body's fight-or-flight response to stress. If stress persists, mental and physical health are undermined, partly because the stress hormones, adrenaline and cortisol, interfere with functioning of the circulatory and immune systems. Relaxation combats many of these effects.

Response to Stress

- Adrenaline is released into bloodstream; heart rate and blood pressure increase
- Liver releases energy, stored as glycogen; blood-sugar and cholesterol levels increase
- Faster breathing; increased metabolic rate
- Muscular tension; increased production of lactic acid
- Gastric acid increases or decreases; digestive enzymes and inhibited peristals is increased
- Perspiration increases
- Increased levels of cortisol; immune system inhibited
- Emotional tension, as attention is focused on emergency reaction

Long-Term Effects of Stress

- High blood pressure; anxiety; insomnia; irritability
- High cholesterol levels

- Breathlessness; hyperventilation; palpitations
- Muscular aches and pains, including headaches and backpain
- Nausea; indigestion; constipation; ulcers; food intolerances
- Skin rashes; eczema
- Raised cortisol levels increase the risk of problems in the immune system
- Emotional outbursts; depression
- Responses to relaxation
- Decreased adrenaline levels; lower blood pressure; less stress on cardiovascular system, decreased blood sugar and cholesterol levels, slower breathing improved lung function and metabolic rate
- Relaxed muscles less lactic acid in muscles
- Improved digestive process
- Improved physiological stability
- Increased activity of immune system; less susceptibility to illness
- Emotional calm; increased alertness and energy.

□□□□

14.
PANCH PRANA–SUB–DIVISIONS OF PRANA

These are also called 'Pancha Pranas', that is Prana, Apana, Samana, Udana and Vyana. Now, a brief description of the five sub-Pranas.

Prana Vayu

Its field of action is entered around and on heart. It also affects mouth, tongue, throat, nose, eyes and skin. Prana Vayu exerts control over life. Force, heart, mind, salivation, spitting, vomiting, eructations, process of respiration, cough, and also helps to let in food. Vitiation of this vayu causes hiccough and respiratory problems.

Udana Vayu

It is seated in the throat, but also exerts its influence upon nose, throat, thorax and umbilicus. It causes and promotes desire/tendency to speak, sing, swallow etc. Its vitiation can cause disorders related to collar bone, larynx (voice box or organ), mouth infections, stammering, dumbness etc.

Samana Vayu

It is centred around the navel, but also moves to pubic area and stomach. Its main function lies in promoting digestion, providing requisite aid to quicken the process of food digestion and to segregate juices, faecal matter and urine from the indigestion food-stuff. Its vitiation causes loose motions, colitis, indigestion, wind/gas trouble etc.

Apana Vayu

Its field of action is quite wide as it relates to digestive system, including anus, bladder, seminal duct, testicles, pubic region. It helps to facilitate expulsion of faeces, urine, semen, menstrual flow and foetus. When Apana Vayu gets vitiated, obstruction is created in the process of expulsion of the said objects. If Apana Vayu is in order, all other types of Vayu are also in perfect order.

Vyana Vayu

This type of Vayu pervades all over the body and controls motions eye-lids, lips, tongue, hands, feet, fingers, genitalia, anus etc. If this Vayu gets vitiated paralysis of single part or whole body takes place. It also must not be forgotten in case of tension, convulsion, retarded mobility etc.

In addition to the above, there are five minor or Up a Pranas:

i) Naga - Responsible for hiccuping and belching

ii) Koorma - It opens the eyes

iii) Krikara - It induces thirst and hunger

iv) Devadatta - It is responsible for yawning

v) Dhanajaya - It is responsible for the decomposition of the body after death.

□□□□

15.
SCIENTIFIC WAY OF BREATHING

Prana means the vital force or life energy and means to control. Hence, pranayama means to control the vital energy by control of breath or the breathing process. But the question arises what is prana? What is the need of regulation of prana and what are its benefits?

The breathing process goes on in the body, since birth till death. The process of inhaling air and exhaling is called breathing. Prana is that inner energy, that is present in all animate and inanimate matter. Hence, the air, we breathe, is different from the prana. Air, we take in, has a gross form, while prana has a subtle form.

The two bases of this creation are–akaga (ether) and prana (vital life force). Both are omnipresent. The vibrance of the vital life force in the ether led to creation. Prana or vital life force is, thus, said to be before the creation of the mind.

The scriptures have elucidated the practice of pranayama for controlling the mind. Prana is the omnipresent vital life force that energises and spurs the mind. We take in prana through the breath. Taking a deep breath fills the three parts of lungs with pranic energy. These three parts are the upper part upto the neck, the parts on both sides of the heart and lower parts. Besides this, the pranic energy even starts to flow to the navel region, when we take deep breath. If we do not inhale-exhale, properly, or if we do not perform pranayama, these parts remain deprived of the vital energy. Through the blood, pranic energy is transferred to all parts of the body. Following are some verses from the ancient texts, elucidate the importance of pranic energy.

The Rigveda States -

All living beings that live from the mountains to the ocean, breathe air in two ways only–inhale and exhale. If these are mastered, then all the six sense-organs will work, harmoniously.

After mastering postures, by retention of inhalation and exhalation, one should practice the science of breathing called pranayama.

In fact, all ancient Indian texts, like the Vedas and the Smrtis, elucidate the importance of pranayama.

There are seven centres in the human body, through which the pranic energy is transferred into the various parts of the body. These centres are called chakras, i.e., psychic centres. If even one chakra is in a state of imbalance, the body is stricken by some ailment or the other. Pranayama is important for bringing up and maintaining this balance. In spiritual terms, it is the path to total emanciation.

Although in this physical body, the pranic energy is in one form, but, according to the different activities in the body, the prana divides itself into five main divisions. These are called pailca pranas. There are further five sub-divisions of prana, called the pailca upapranas.

The five divisions are prana, apana, samana, udana and vyana, while the sub-divisions are naga, kurma, krikala, devadatta, dhananjaya.

The age, to which a human being can be expected to live, can be determined by the pranic energy, derived by him through breathing. Those who breathe shallow and quick live a shorter life span in comparison to those who breathe, deep and slow. The ancients studied the different animals and came to this conclusion. As snakes, elephants and tortoises have a slow rate of breathing, they have a longer life span. While animals like dogs, rabbits and birds which have a fast breathing rate are short-lived. Hence, through pranayama, one cannot just have physical and spiritual benefits, rather one could enhance one's life span. The following table would show how the rate of breathing has a direct effect on one's life span.

1.	Tortoise	4-5 times per minute life span - 200 Years
2.	Snake	7-8 times per minute life span - 150 years
3.	Man	15-16 times a minute life span - 100 years
4.	Horse	20-22 times a minute life span - 40 years
5.	Dog	28-30 times a minute life span - 14 years

The text, Svara Yoga, explains what the effect would be when the exhaled air is thrown out at a certain distance. Normally, in rechaka or exhalation, the breath, coming out, can be felt at a distance of twelve finger from the nostrils. While puraka or inhalation can be felt ten finger away. If the recka is felt 11 fingers away, then, the pranic energy gets stabilized; 10 fingers, one gets peace and happiness; 9 fingers, one becomes a poet; 8 fingers, one becomes eloquent; 7 finger breadths, one becomes foresighted; 6 finger breadths, one becomes capable of flying in the sky; 5 fingers, one can travel at the speed of thought; 4 fingers, one gains the eight siddhis or spiritual powers (supra) normal powers; 3 fingers, one comes to possess the nine nidhis, i.e., treasures or the keys to worldly prosperity; 2 fingers, one becomes capable of assuming several physical forms at the same time; I finger, one can become invisible; 1/10 of I fingers, one conquers death.

In different activities, rechka has the following force -

normal state	-	upto six fingers
emotional state	-	upto 12 fingers

singing	-	upto 16 fingers
eating	-	upto 20 fingers
walking	-	upto 24 fingers
sleeping	-	upto 30 fingers
sexual activity and exercising	-	36 fingers

All this explanation has been given to make one understand the importance of pranayama. One can control the speed and depth of the breathing for physical and spiritual gains.

It is through the prana, i.e., the vital life force, that one can form a link between the body and the soul. Hence, prana is the link between the gross and the subtle world. A body, without prana, is usually declared dead and one could say that the soul has left for the heaven.

First of all, pranayama keeps the body healthy and, secondly, it keeps the mind, still and concentrated. If the pranic energy keeps flowing, continuously and unhindered, through the susumna channel related to kundalini, then, the path to spiritual progress opens up for the person. Pranayama also increases the sexual power, Through celibacy, pure-balanced diet and pranyama, one could enhance one's mental powers, as well. Through pranayama, even though restricted by the medium of this small physical form, being in this physical body, one can possess all the divine powers of the universe, as it is, and also, in their true form.

Pranayama affects the entire body system and tones the blood circulation, glandular system, nervous system, pranic energy channel network, the store of pranic energy in the body and the subtle body.

□□□□

16.
SOME IMPORTANT GUIDELINES FOR PRANAYAMA

- One should practise pranayama in an airy, open, well-ventilated place. One should not practise it in a room filled with dust, smoke, dampness, bad odour and rubbish. One should, also not try in very fast blowing wind.
- One should try on an empty stomach or four hours after meals or half an hour before meals.
- One should wear clothes according to the season but they should not be very tight.
- It is best to practise early in the morning. In winters, one could also try at noon or in the evening.
- Practise pranayama after yoga postures and before meditation.
- During pranayama, keep the body relaxed and loose.
- Sit on a folded blanket, covered with a cotton cloth, for pranayama. Sit in any meditative pose.
- One can practise more during winters than summers.
- Do not practise bhastrika and suryabhedi, during summers. In winters, refrain from practising sitali, sitkari and chandrabhedi pranayamas.
- Those suffering from asthma, high blood pressure, hypertension and heart problems should not practise kumbhaka without the proper guidance of an expert.

- Do not put extra force on the body, during pranayama. Hold the breath, only as long as it is comfortable. Otherwise, it might create an adverse effect on the lungs.
- Those practising pranayama, should avoid smoking, tobacco, meat and alcohol.
- Those with wind humour predominant should not practise and those with bile humour dominant should not practise suryabhedi and those with phlegm predominant should not practise chandrabhedi pranayama.
- Suryabhedi cures imbalance of wind, humour, ujjaya cures phlegm imbalance, Sitali and Sitkari cure bile imbalance while Mastrika cures the imbalance of all the three.
- One should practise asanas after having a bath. Otherwise, one should bathe half an hour after the practice.
- If one starts sweating, instead of wiping it off with a towel, one should massage with the hands and dry it off or let it dry off, naturally.
- If one is suffering from cold or the nostrils are blocked, then, one should not practise pranayama.
- One should not break the practice, again and again. Otherwise, the benefits cannot be attained, fully, and will not last long.

For the practice of pranayama, one should understand the breathing process, properly. Breathing can be of two types abdominal breathing and chest breathing.

Udara Svasana (Abdominal Breathing)

Lie down on the floor on your back like the corpse-pose and place one hand's palm on the navel. Inhale deeply in a way that the abdomen bellows like a balloon and rises. The more the navel region rises the diaphragm goes down. Diaphragm is the tissue wall that separates the lungs from the abdomen.

Next, exhale slowly. For this, contract the abdomen and allow the hand on the navel to go downwards, rather push it towards the spine. As the abdominal region contracts, the chest expands. Keep the chest and shoulders still during the practice. Repeat 10 to 15 times.

Urah Savasana (Chest Breathing)

Sit with crossed legs or lie down. Expanding the chest, breathe in deeply. If necessary, place the hands on the waist with the thumbs positioned on the back, while the rest of the fingers on your stomach and, then, with the rest of the fingers, press the stomach in.

Exhale i.e. perform rechaka, allowing the chest to sink in. Inhale i.e. perform puraka, allowing only the chest to expand. In this practice, do not expand or contract the stomach. Repeat 5 to 10 times.

Both the above practices are very good for the health of any person. Generally, as one is not able to breathe, deeply, in this manner in the normal course. These preparatory practices of pranayama are necessary for good health and longevity too.

Purna Svasana or Yogic Svasana (Yogic Breathing)

Sitting in any comfortable posture raise the hands above the head and place the arms on the back from above the shoulders. Push back the elbows by your head. Thus, the ribs will be stretched and the chest will expand to the maximum. Expanding both the chest and the abdomen, fill the lungs with air, performing paraka. After this, relaxing the abdomen and the chest, perform recaka or exhale. In the end, by pressing the abdomen and contracting the chest, expel all the air present in the lungs. The entire practice should be rhythmic and not in jerks.

Pranayama is described in two parts here, (a) Preparatory practices of pranayama, (b) Pranayama.

□□□□

17.
PRANAYAMA
– THE METHODS AND MEANING

By the term Pranayama is meant regulation of Prana and its distribution to various parts of the body. Pranayama is performed by

i) Manipulation of respiration beyond its normal limit. (H) Stretching it.

ii) Flowing it down so as to experience the full range of respiration of gross and subtle levels.

Pranayama is Performed By Following Methods

- By inhaling the breath in quick succession and then exhaling.
- By inhaling Prana (air or life energy) by one nostril and exhalation through the other.
- By inhalation of Prana through both the nostrils, retain the same as person's capacity and then releasing the same gradually, until the stomach is fully emptied.
- While inhaling the stomach should inflate and lungs contract or squeeze.
- While exhaling stomach should get drawn in or squeezed and lungsexpanded.
- Quick respiration, resembling bellow of a black smith.

- By throwing out prana forcefully and then inhaling the same.
- By sudden stoppage or suspension of breath and then retaining the residual part there of within the body as per one's capacity.

During meditation normal breathing should be maintained and mind should be concentrated upon breathing and wayward thoughts should be controlled. To perform Pranayama an aspirant can sit in any convenient asana (sitting posture) like Padmasana, Swastikasana, Siddhasana or simply squat on the floor, bed or even sit in a chair or sofa, as an inconvenient posture will not allow your mind to concentrate.

Rhythmic Respiration (Breathing)

In natural breathing no discomfort is felt, and natural/normal breathing is another nomeclation of rhythmic breathing which differs in case of every person.

Variations in Breathing Process

i) Irregular breathing indicates tension.

ii) Shallow and rapid breathing is indicative of anxiety.

iii) Forceful and short breathing means state of anger.

iv) Relaxed state of body and mind indicates a rhythmic, slow and smooth respiration.

v) Gasping and arrhythmic breathing indicates a state of grief.

vi) When there is irregular breathing, it indicates disturbed mental states and neurosis.

vii) Breathing can even be incomplete and uneven in certain types of neurosis.

viii) Slow rhythmic breathing is believed to impact and create feelings of relaxation, reduced muscle tension and alpha brain waves.

To begin with, try to tune into the rhythms of breath and align the same with the outside world. This, invariably, includes, heart beat, brain rhythms, mental emotional, emotive (emotional) and mental rhythms, wakefulness and sleep etc. but there are always variations in intensity and frequency. All such rhythms occur in relation to changes in weather conditions, mental states, seasons, months, years, and planetory influences. Generally, we are not aware of presence of rhythmic force within our body and mind but Pranayama leads and helps us to realise such rhythmic forces. Constant and regular practice of pranayama can help us to know the changes occurring within the body and also know as to where we are lacking and where improvement is required. A trained mind can help to control such mechanisms so that areas of consciousness and control, (which are generally not within our control) can be unravelled.

Kriyas During Pranayama

Following terms are often used in relation to inhalation, retention and expulsion/release/exhalation of breath (Prana).

1. POORAK KRIYA : Process of inhalation.
2. KUMBHAK KRIYA: To retain or control.
3. RECHAK KRIYA : Exhalation of breath.

If prana/vayu is inhaled but not exhaled, suffocation, laboured breathing, choking may be felt. Hence any breath that is inhaled has to be exhaled so as to avoid discomforts. Moreover, after quick succession of inhalation and exhalation, gap is necessary so as to relax the overworked organs. One has to keep balance between inhaled and exhaled air or Prana, as deficient inspiration will not suffice to nurture the body as a whole and excessive inspiration will overtax our system.

Yogic postures are not simply physical exercises, they are much more than that–they ensure and fortify mental tendencies, faculties, provide succour to your agitated mind and nerves and strengthen your body. Due to space crunch, it is not possible to give a detailed account of all faces of yoga which is science in itself. These are neither physical exercises nor body building devices, nor modern health clubs, health points, gyms, slimming and weight-loss clinics nor are they source of delight for the elite or pseudo rich classes, they are meant to purify body and mind, provide alacrity, suppleness, agility, peace and tranquillity to mind, to divert the body from diseased states and also to impart immunity from diseases and infections, to arouse body's defence mechanisms.

Pranayama

Pranayama literally means pause during respiration but actually it means control over inhalation and exhalation process. It is the only method by which you can quite easily tone up your entire body, regulate circulation of blood, normalise respiration, increase your heart-beats as also slow down cardiac rhythm by sheer control, let blood reach even the minutest blood vessels and, above all, it requires minimal effort. Pranayarna also brings under control your wayward thoughts, keeps you away from worry and tension, imparts sobriety and tranquility to your agitated temperament.

The readers should go through this chapter carefully and, after studying the same, they would find that most of their mental and physical problems have been addressed to and solved. So, without categorising or nomeclating a particular disease and its causative symptom(s) an easy, but effective way, has been suggested. Pranayama has been dealt with under the following 8 classifications, viz.

1. Suryabhedi
2. Ujjayi,
3. Sitkari,
4. Shitali.
5. Bhastrika,
6. Bharamari,
7. Moorchha, and
8. Plavini.

Three terms would be quite frequently used here. Inhalation (Rechaka), Suspension or withholding (Kumbhak) and Release (Poorak) of breath.

□□□□

18.
PRANAYAMA
– ITS HEALING POWER & BENEFITS

The breath which enters our body from without (outside) is called 'Shwas' or inhalation of air, and that which goes out from our body is called exhalation or 'Prashawas'. Breath is the life force or vital force or, still better, the sustaining force of our body. Proper balance between inhalation, retention and exhalation forms the very basis of our life (jeevan). Death is nothing other than existence of this process. It is also subtly called 'Prana'. Pranayama is divided into three stages.

1. Poorak : The terms implies inhalation of air (breath) or inspiration.
2. Kumbhak : It means withholding of breath.
3. Rechak : The term is indicative of exhalation of breath.

Procedure of Pranayama

It is, in fact, a practice for complete respiration. Sit in Padmasana or Sukhasana. Keep your spinal cord erect. Inhale fresh air through the nose, filling your abdomen with the air. When the abdomen is full (by inhalation of air) and bloates, retain the breath as long as you can, without suffocating choking, tiring or straining yourself. Now slowly exhale the air. While inhaling the lungs would contract and the abdomen bloat but when air is exhaled, the abdomen will squeeze and lungs expand. Entire process is called respiratory process. Ratio between all the three stages (Poorak, Kumbhak and Rechak) should preferably be 1:2:1 but there are no hard and fast rules guidelines. Pranayama can be done even while you are walking, moving on foot or in a vehicle, sitting in a chair (preferably) easy chair, lying down or standing. The only common factor of utmost importance being that the air inhaled must be fresh and pure. If Pranayama done in a choked, smoky, dusty, polluted and toxic environs, it will cause harm, and there is no wonder you may expose your body to various serious disorders.

The Two Naris

Our nose has two nostrils, the left one is called 'Chandra Nari' and the right one is called 'Surya Nari'. One denotes cool and the other heat, one is active at night while the other is active during the day. When we inhale the breath is cold but, when exhale, it is hot. There are certain ascities who can easily forecast death time of a person from the determination of breathing process, time and speed of breathing as, after all, it is the breath which is the vital force of our moods, climatic changes, etc. Lunar and solar phases and eclipses affect changes in nature, world events, lives of all persons, etc. First of all breath through one nostril only, closing the other with the index finger of your hand. Now retain the breath as long and as conveniently you can. There after, slowly breath out the finger. Before you exhale, the nostril, through which you had breathed should be closed. After a reasonable pause, now follow the same process from the other nostril. Inhalation and breathing processes should be slow and uniform.

Benefits of Pranayama

As already discussed, pranayma aims at fortifying, sustaining and nurturing vital force of the body. It is connected more with our mental faculties than physical. It corrects various, if not all, physical disorders, by training the mind in such a way that body is rendered strong enough to take the oddities and abnormalities of life and other upsets in normal way, and upheavals and disturbances fail to have any impact on body. It removes defects and abnormalities of eyes, senses of hearing, smell, touch, speech, and purifies blood, normalises breathing process, tones up digestive organs, improves appetite, activates functioning of secretary glands, retards old age, takes away all evil feelings, recharges mental faculties. Above all, it provides peace (mental), sense of satisfaction, happiness and bliss. This is an asana to improve your life span. Recharge your emotions and other activities, by doing it regularly.

Kinds of Pranayama

There are eight kinds of Pranayama viz.

1. Surya-Bhedan
2. Ujjayi,
3. Sitkari
4. Shitali
5. Bhastrika
6. Bhramari
7. Moorchha and
8. Plavini. –Hereunder, brief description and benefits of each Kriya are described -

Surya-Bhedan

It pertains to performing pranayama through the Surya-Nari (Right Nostril). Sit in Padma, Sidha or Swatikasana. Inhale fresh air through the right nostril, closing the left nostril (Chandra Nari) with your index finger. Inhaled breath should be suspended or retained as far and as long as possible. Before suffocation sets in, breath out through the left nostril, keeping your index finger on the right nostril. The trinity of Poorak, Kumbhak and Rechak should be done without any discomfort.

Benefits - It is highly useful, particularly in winter. It improves appetite, purifies blood and respiratory system, imparts agility and suppleness to body, sharpens and purifies memory, gives a feeling of freshness, imparts glow and lustre to body, dispels mental and physical fatigue. Both men and women of all ages are advised to do this Pranayama daily but more particularly in winter to let the body get vital heat.

Ujjayi

Sit in Padma, Sidha or Swatikasana (whichever suits you as the most comfortable and easy). Expel forcibly the air from the body. While expelling breath, there must be the sound which is heard during sleep, as if you are expelling air during sleep. Thereafter, inhale fresh air to the full capacity of your lungs, expanding your chest as far as you can. In this pranayma, breath is not to be retained. When you feel lungs are fully filled with air release/breath out the air slowly, making sure that during the course of expelling air, there is natural own of exhalation process.

Benefits - The process can be done while walking, writing, sitting, getting up. It modifies heat (excessive) in the body, improves secretion of digestive juices, increases appetite, removes constipation, cough and other respiratory disorders. Also provides lustre to the body. It should be performed daily by people of both sexes, irrespective of age.

Sitkari

Be seated in Swastika, Padma or Sidha asana. Let your tongue stay in-between both the rows of teeth. Now slightly clinch your teeth but very gently and softly, so that tongue is not unduly put under pressure of the teeth, both rows should simply touch the tongue so that it does not slip or retrace. Keep your lips open. Now take a deep breath through the mouth, creating a 'hissing' sound (the soul as created by a snake). Retain the breath as far as feasible. Thereafter exhale through the nose very slowly.

Benefits - This exercise is highly beneficial during hot days as it not only dispels ill effects of heat but imparts cooling effect to the body. It modifies excessive bile, improves appetite, dispels lethargy and renders body beautiful. Does not let teeth decay and also promotes general health and texture of teeth. It also induces natural and own sleep. Ladies can also perform this asana.

Shitali

Lengthwise twist the tongue in the form of a crow's beak (or resembling a crow's beak) and slightly protrude the tongue out of lips. Now breathe in through the tongue. Retain the breath by closing your mouth. Do not allow breath to escape out. Before a suffocating tendency surfaces, exhale fully the breath and relax.

Benefits - It is almost a panacea for all types of fever. Also cures all the stomach disorders. All men and women can do it.

Bhastrika

Be seated in a comfortable position (whether in Sidha Padma or Padma asana). Now inhale through both the nostrils in the same way as air in the willow of a black-smith is filled in and eased out. Breathing in and breathing out process, must create an identical sound as comes from the willow. While drawing in breath, your belly should bloat but, while blowing out, your belly should squeeze. Whenever you feel suffocated, exhale through the right nostril. Now repeat the process through the left nostril other process remaining unchanged. Entire process should be done in alteration.

Benefits - Yogis perform this process to awaken Kundalini. It activates digestive juices, thereby arousing natural appetite, removes disorders of the three humours (wind, bile and phlegm), cures and rectifies all throat diseases, does away with cough and asthma, imparts strength and energy to heart and regulated functioning thereof, modifies and normalises pulmonary, respiratory processes improves circulation of blood by activating blood vessels.

Bhramari

Sit in Sidha, Padma or Swastikasana, keeping your spine erect. Inhale through the left nostril, while inhalation create sound like that of a big black bee (Bhramara). Retain breath as long and as you conveniently can. Thereafter slowly exhale through the right nostril.

Benefits - It clears obstruction in the nose, removes heavy feeling in the head, facilitates breathing through nose, pacifies wayward mental attitudes, keeps mind under happiness and transquillity. It will calm down and pacify mental agitation, if performed daily in the evening.

Moorchha

This should be performed while sitting in a sidhasana as it is a bit difficult posture. Before deciding to practically perform this asana, it is imperative that full guidance is sought from a yoga expert, otherwise it can do more harm than good. Only those, whether ladies or gents, who are desirous to perform it, should have a strong will to follow the rigid norms and follow the complexities before harping on the process. Relevant process is detailed hereunder.

First of all, be seated in Siddhasana. Take a deep breath through both the nostrils. Now retain in the breath, your chin rested on the hollow position of throat (as is done in a Jalandhar Bhandha). Two fingers close to your thumbs (index and middle fingers) of both hands should be delicately placed and rested on your both eyes (over the upper lids). Keep both eyes closed (right eye, with right hand fingers and left eye with left hand fingers). Place the four fingers of both hands on either side of each nose, thus closing both the nostrils. Now the small fingers should be placed just below the lower left, lifting the lower lip so that the same is raised so much that it joins the upper lip (that is when mouth is closed with the help of two little fingers). Now apply the process of 'Mool Bandh' (by stretching your anus and rectum upwards) and 'Udyan Bandha'. Before you start suffocating, release and remove the fingers and exhale through both the nostrils.

Benefits - It pacifies wayward mind, helps in concentrating mind, removes diseases pertaining to blood, skin and respiration. It preserves semen, all stomach and digestive problems disappear. There is no night discharge. Digestion improves, body is infused with extra energy. Mool Bandha helps to awaken the kundalini. It is not recommended for ladies.

Plavini

Sit in Padmasana and inhale (fresh) air so that stomach is filled to its filling capacity. Bloat your abdomen as much as you can. Now exhale the breathe. This process be repeated 4-5 times. Before you breathe in again, make sure that your abdomen contracts completely after you have exhaled.

Benefits - Renders the entire body supple and light, cleans the bowels in such a way that digestion stands improved, disorders like pile, gas accumulation, extra fat from and around abdomen is shed. It improves figure of a person in general. It is claimed that any person who becomes an adopt in this process may float over water like a lotus, swim or even walk on the water, even if turbulent.

Breathing exercises

Breathing with rhythm. Sit cross-legged on the ground or on a chair or stand with folded hand as in prayer. Keep mouth closed and breathe in through the nostrils counting one to four. Hold breath till you count from one to eight. Start to breathe out. While breathing out count once again from one to four, hold breath till you count from five to eight before you start inhaling. Repeat this a few more times. Increase the number of counts while breathing in and out and in between, gradually from day to day, to draw in more oxygen and expel more carbon-dioxide.

Cleansing Pranayama

Sit cross-legged on the ground or on a chair with the spine erect and muscles relaxed. Cover the right nostril with the thumb and inhale through the left nostril. Cover the left nostrils too with the index finger and hold breath for one to two counts. Release the thumb and exhale through the right nostril. Repeat this with the left nostril. Cover the left nostril with the index finger and inhale rough the right. Close both the nostrils and hold for one or two counts and then exhale through the left nostril releasing the index finger. With regular practice the number of counts while holding the breath should increase.

This exercise corrects the disorders of the nasal cavity and lungs. The good supply of oxygen help purify the lungs.

Those who suffer from blood pressure must not practice to hold the breath. They can simply inhale and exhale.

One other exercise - Sit in a comfortable position with crossed legs. Keep the body relaxed and erect. Keep the mouth closed. Inhale fast as much air as possible and exhale quickly with force. Do not hold the breath but breathe in and out in quick succession. Relax a while, breathing normally and again start breathing in and out in quick succession. Do this five to six times in the beginning and slowly increase after a few days practice.

This exercise is recommended in all digestive and respiratory disorders. It corrects defective circulation.

□□□□

19.
SCIENCE OF CHANTING – JAPA YOGA

This is the best means of purification of the mind. Although it is harder than prarthana (prayer), yet, if done with tapasya (penance), it proves quick in producing result. Japa means repeating a powerful spiritual word. Repeating a particular word in the mind for progress on the path of attaining oneness with the Supreme Being or Brahman (the all-pervading self) is called japa-yoga. For this, two things are important–the mantra, to be chanted and the mala i.e., rosary, to keep count of the chantings.

Mantra, a syllable, is not an ordinary word or group of words. Rather, it is extraordinary and, through its resonance, the deep-rooted tendencies and passions are banished. Mantra is a group of words instilled with the powers of some. Hence, it is better to get a mantra from a guru (master). The best mantra for an aspirant is one which is in perfect harmony with his soul and which awakens devotion in him. There are infinite mantras, pertaining to the different gods, goddesses and deities in different religions and sects. Hence, it is best to ask the guru which mantra would suit one and, then, one should get diksha (spiritual initiation in a particular mantra-practice) from the guru.

A mala i.e., rosary has 108 beads. Each bead is secured with a knot which represents the worldly bonds and is called brahmagranthi. Other than the 108 beads, there is one more, which is tied separately, to the main string of the rosary. It is called sumeru. It helps in keeping a tab on the number of rounds of the rosary. There are rosaries with 11, 21, 27, 33, 36 and 54 beads for special purposes. Rosaries, with beads of rudraksa (seed of a sacred tree), sphatika (rock-crystal), etc., are used for different purposes.

There can be four types of japa–likhita (written), vaikhari (oral), upaihgu (murmuring) and manasika (mental). Those with a very fickle and restless mind should practice likhita japa. To write the mantra in beautiful handwriting on a page with a feeling of devotion and love for one's deity is called likhita japa. When, through this type of japa, the senses become calm and concentrated, then, one should start vaikhari japa. In vaikhari japa, one should sit in a meditative pose and relax the mind and the body. Then, one should close the eyes and forming the image of the deity in one's mind, one should chant the mantra, clearly and loudly. But this should be practised alone in the room. One should concentrate on the resonance of the mantra. This is called vaikhari japa.

Then, seated as before, if one chants the mantra silently, murmuring in such a way that the mantra can be heard only by himself and not even by a person sitting beside, is called upansu japa. Silent chanting does not mean that one can get away with incorrect pronunciation. Rather, it means that if someone else is in the room he or she should be able to see your lips moving but not hear the mantra. The last is manasika japa. In it, one is to sit as before but one should chant the mantra in the mind without even moving the lips or tongue and keeping the mouth shut. This is the best method of chanting.

The preliminary aspirants should practise likhita japa. A little advanced category of aspirants could practise the other three types. (1) those capable of only vaikhari japa; (2) those capable of both vaikhari and upanshu japas; and (3) those who chant one round of vaikhari, two rounds upaighu and three rounds manasika. The highest category of aspirants, i.e., adepts for elephant practise only manasika japa.

By chanting a mantra daily right from the day one, you get it from the Master, unto the time of death, is called nitya japa, eternal or obligatory chant. Chanting a certain number in a certain period of days, as directed by the mantra, is called anusthana. The highest form of anusthana is called purascarana, which is quite tough.

Rules for the Chanting of Mantras

- The rosary should not be seen by others. Hence, it should be held in the hand, inside a cloth pouch, called gomukhi.
- One should not cross the sumeru the 109th bead, when moving the beads.
- One should not touch the forefinger and the little finger to the rosary.
- Pronunciation of the mantra should be clear and correct.
- The speed of chanting should be constant so that it is in rhythm.
- Chanting should be done without any desire.
- Do not reveal the mantra to anyone.
- One should choose a particular spot, a particular sitting posture a particular cotton or woolen piece of cloth or blanket and a particular time, daily, for the chanting.
- It is more effective to chant the mantra, facing the north or east.
- Keep concentrating on the meaning of the mantra and the deity, whom one is worshipping while chanting the mantra. It is said in the text Patanjali Yoga-Sutra (1/27).

The mind is clouded by three obstacles on the path of Yoga restlessness, impurity and foolishness. The aim of japa is to free the mind of these three. When the mind is pure, then, it becomes capable of realising the soul.

Ajapa - Japa (Non-Stop Eternal Chanting)

To keep repeating the mantra is called japa. The japa becomes ajapa, when the mantra gets repeated in the mind on its Ajapa-japa goes on, subconsciously, all the time, while japa is consciously.

Ajapa-japa is a complete sadhana (spiritual practice) in it. If this starts and one becomes aware of it, then, one can enter into the state of meditation, i.e., dhyana. This type of japa helps in banishing passions, desires and fears and makes the very pure. When there is an explosion of the latent passion tendencies, one should not react. Rather, one should just watch them like an audience. Otherwise, these passions can lead to spiritual downfall. This type of japa also frees the mind and body of all ailments and weaknesses.

Generally, "soham" mantra is used for this purpose, but other mantra also can be used.

In the beginning, i.e., first stage, the aspirant should concentrate on the breathing. He should practise this meditative pose. Breathe in and feel the chest and abdomen region, becoming empty. After concentrating on the breath for sometime, in the second stage, feel the resonance of the same, while inhaling, and, hum, when exhaling. Do this for breath. After one month of practice, reverse the process.

In second stage first breathe out and feel the resonance and, then, breathing in, and feel the resonance of so. In words, in the second stage, *chant hamso.*

In the third stage, *chant so hamso.*

In the fourth stage, continuously, chant mentally only s *soham* so that there is no break between so and ham.

Pratyahara

In the fifth stage, chant, mentally, performing khechari-mudra and ujjayi pranayama.

In the sixth stage, move the conscience on the chakras of the kundalini. If possible, continue to be aware of the resonance and try to concentrate the prana on each chakra. In the last stage, one becomes a witness to what was happening in the earlier stages. One has to be fully conscious, in this stage, and not fall asleep.

When a person is able to continue in the final stage he enters into the highest level of meditation and, then, into samadhi.

Precautions and Guidelines

Practise withdrawal of senses, one by one, beginning with the most turbulent one and this has to be done, gently not vehemently. Detach your mind from its desired objects. The best way is to withdraw the senses, too, along with prana, which is the cause of action. You have to be alert and vigilant in annihilating all desires with the sword of dispassion and the axe of discrimination. For this, one cannot do on one's accord, so guru and God's grace are essential. For that, devotion and surrender are the tools.

Observance of silence, moderation in diet, steadiness in pose, dispassion, regularity in the practice of asana and pranayama, patience, contentment, perseverance, tenacity, celibacy, seclusion, discrimination between the real and the non-real are all aids to pratyahara.

The obstacles to pratyahara are passions and desires, too much working, too much mixing with worldly people, too much worldly activity, too much food, too much walking, too much curiosity in external affairs, slackness and laziness in practices, etc. Every practitioner should be careful about one's own wavery mind and recognise by self-analysis which quality is dominant in him. Accordingly, one has to decide the practices that he has to adopt and way of life that he has to lead to attain salvation, at the earliest.

20.
AURA – A LUMINOUS CLOUD

The idea of a human aura, a relating luminous cloud surrounding the body is an ancient one. It became so popular in Christian art before the aura was considered an attribute of ordinary everyday morals. For centuries, it has been believed that clairvoyant people could actively see an aura surrounding ordinary visuals, and this aura differed from person to person in colour and character, expressing the health, emotional and spiritual attributes of the subject. The visionary Swedenborg wrote in his spiritual diray, "There is a spiritual sphere surrounding everyone as well as a natural and corporeal our."

There are 3 major sources of Prana

i) Solar Prana

ii) Air Prana and

iii) Ground Prana

Five elements that compose human body are Air, Heat, Earth, Vacuum and Water and the classifications, as shown above, engulf there of the five elements. To keep our body alive we need life energy (Prana or Ki'). It is known as a 'Pneuma' (in Greek) 'Mana'(In Poynesian) and 'Ruah'(the Hebrew) which means "the breath of life". In order to rid the patient of his illness, the healer projects the health of life (Prana or Ki) to him. This type of Prana healing is also called 'Miraculous Healing', though there may not seem any miracle in this process.

Solar Prana

It is derived from sunlight and is utilized to promote good health by invigorating the body. One can obtain the solar energy of drinking water exposed in the sun or by sunbathing or even by taking bath in the sun or massaging the body under the sunlight. Since solar energy is extremely potent, the patient must expose his body to the sun to Solar Prana. Certain persons have hypersensitive and tender skin, hence they must be extra cautions while exposing their bodies. Persons having bilious tendency ought to be overcautious.

Air Prana

It is an air vitatity globe (Air Prana) which is absorbed by the lungs through breathing as also absorbed directly by the bioplasmic body's energy centres. More volume/quantity of Air Prana can be better absorbed deep, slow, and rhythmic breathing than by short, rapid and shallow breathing. Certain well trained experts can absorb less energy through the skin pores.

Ground Prana

It is also called 'ground vitality globe' which is ăbsorbed through soles of the feet (by walking barefoot). It is also absorbed unnoticed, unconsciously or automatically. If one can draw in ground prana to enhance one's vitality, ability to think more correctly, capacity to more work, one should learn to exhausted ground Prana consciouly.

So far, only such factors have been described which help the life energy to activate the diseased organs. First, we have to activate and energise the blocked passages because, as long as such inhibiting factors are not removed, prana energy cannot reach the body, and more particularly to the diseased organs. If the ailment is too chronic and complicated, one has to, naturally, spend more tune to remove the bottleneck. A healer must know which organ is to be energized and what among of life energy is actually needed to affect proper cure. The healer and the patient have to exert patience and perserverance, as there is no room for a complacent approach or half-baked treatment. Further , mental disorders may take more time to cure the physical disorders, though direct relationship between mind and physical body cannot be denied.

□□□□

21.
INNER VISUALIZATION – ANTAH DARSHAN

In antah darsana (the inner visualization), one has to visualize all the events and actions, that took place outside, in day or night time in the mind, like a dream. But one should not fall asleep and one should be aware that this witnessing is not actually a dream but a conscious effort. In this practice, one has to recall and visualize all the important events and actions, involved in it, right from the time of waking up, in the morning to the time of lying down to sleep.

You have to visualize exactly all details like going to a friend's place, the exact location of his house, the vehicle you used and the people you saw. Or, you could recall going to the temple, the priest, who greeted you, the various utensils kept there, the ritual performed there, the worship you performed and the prasada (sweets offered to the Gods), that you got. If you travelled, then, recall the bus or the train you used, the things you saw on the way, the various stations or stops that came on the way and the hustle and bustle, there. You could also recall natural scenes and events, the stars, the sun, the moon which you saw or the different colours and shapes, that you witnessed. If a student, one could recall the scene of one's college or school, one's class, the teacher teaching the class, etc.

In the final stage of this practice, one should pronounce the names of the objects and persons, mentally, that one recalls. This practice increases one's memory and prepares one for further practice.

Cidakasa Darsana
(Cerebral or Conscious Visualization)

The dark and black space that one visualizes in the place of the third eye, i.e., the eyebrow centre, when one closes the eyes is called cidakasa. Concentrating the mind on this spot and, then, visualizing the following types of scenes is called cidakasa darsana.

Sit in a meditative pose. Close the eyes and position the hands in or dhyan-mudra. Concentrate on the sounds around you. Then visualize your own body in the mind. Visualize your physical form seated on the floor. Concentrate the mind on the breathing. Then, concentrate it on th e cidakasa. It has no shape, but if one continues to concentrate, then, after some time, different colours start to appear. Keep viewing them. Now visualize this dark space, not just on the third eye, but all around you, everywhere. One can pronounce the names of the colours one is seeing, mentally. Now, visualize your own form but with a divine radiance in the cidakas. Concentrate on the sound of om, emanating from there. Keep viewing the images that might appear. When ending the practice, perform the reverse, i.e., first, concentrate on the breathing, then, the body and, lastly, on the sounds all around. Then, get up.

Antarmauna (Inner Silence)

Mauna means to be silent outside and inside. In order to reach this state, one shall have to cut oneself off from the commotion outside and restlessness of the mind and the senses. In this practice, a person has an experience of being a witness to everything, which is very important for meditation.

Antarmauna can be divided into three stages: (1) vaksathyama (control of speech); (2) vatig-mauna (silence of speech); and (3) antarmauna (silence of mind, too).

The first stage of antarmauna is called vak-sathyama (control of speech). The eyes, ears and the tongue destroy the peace of the mind and make it tense and worried. Among these three, speech creates most disturbances. Hence, if the speech is controlled, the rest two are controlled on their own. For the practice of vaksathyama, one has to get into the habit of speaking less. For this, remember the following tips do not stress your point too much, speak after due thought, do not get into an argument, do not get involved in criticising others, do not get perturbed by adverse circumstances, do not speak anything that might hurt anyone and, finally, keep your words and voice sweet. Hence, vak-sadhyama means to speak for the good of others, keeping their respect and feelings in mind.

The second stage of antarmauna is vatig-mauna (silence of speech). The ancient texts state–*maunam sarvdrtha sadhanam* (silence is the best way of attaining all wishes). Complete rest of the tongue is called vafig-mauna. When a person is totally silent, the voice of the Lord becomes obvious. This practice increases power of thought, memory and intelligence. Such a person can, then, read the mind of others. Through complete silence, one can know about the restlessness of the mind, the hidden evil tendencies and one's passions. Then, it becomes easy to control them and transform the mind, completely, through the practices, suggested in the ancient texts. An aspirant gains knowledge, divine power and several virtues, like the capability of solving all problems, influencing others through one's speech, etc., because the divine voice works and not his selfish voice.

The third stage of antarmauna can be divided into five substages.

In the first stage, one has to remain aware of the events and the sounds, outside. One should hear and see everything but not react. One has to remain a mere silent witness.

In the second stage, one has to curb the tendency of the eyes and ears to be directed outwards into external objects, i.e., one has to close the eyes and ears and concentrate on the mind, on the thoughts, on its reactions and the various images, being generated in it. Do witness all this but be aware of the self. Be like a witness and do not get involved in the thoughts or the scenario.

In the third stage, go through the first and the second stages, alternatively. In other words, practise outer and inner awareness.

In the fourth stage, sit in a peaceful and isolated place, generate images in the mind and witness them. This practice is called manoraj. These are of two types–natural and artificial. The former is to be avoided and the latter has to be practised. Generally, manorajya is said to be an obstacle on the way to meditation and samadhi, because, in it, a person loses his awareness and becomes completely engrossed and wastes his time. This is natural manorajya here, i.e., in fourth stage too the person does create images in the mind and witnesses them but he does not get involved in them. This is artificial manorajya. In natural manorajya, the aspirant does not create images but, whenever the mind wishes, due to passions, starts to imagine things, he should be aware of it and not get engrossed into it. For this, the aspirant will have to be alert, all the 24 hrs. This is very difficult. Previously, it was mentioned that the former is to be avoided. But, if an adept can practice, being alert all the 24 hours, then, it is not harmful. Such an aspirant gains a capability to curb unnecessary imaginations and be able to utilize the mind's energy, properly and positively. Hence, here, it proves helpful rather than be an obstacle.

In the fifth stage, the mind has to be made totally calm. One has to concentrate on the divine conscience, that is formless. One has to concentrate on divine light. This is a state of stunned silence for the mind. It is like unconsciousness. The difference is that in unconsciousness, the person is not aware of anything but here the person is aware of the state of total silence and also experiences the all-pervading consciousness-existence-bliss.

When the aspirant has perfected this practice, his mind becomes prepared for meditation. Up to now the different techniques were discussed as per the Himalayan tradition. Now, let us see the different techniques as adopted by my master's tradition.

The key to dharana is that, first, you have to recognize your mind, i.e., decide the quality of your mind, then, accordingly, you can choose the object of concentration. Once you start on anything, then you have to avoid the mental confrontation, that will increase the ability of concentration. Relaxation and concentration are interrelated. Therefore, before starting practice perform some relaxation postures, little pranayama, yoga-nidra (little), prarthana and trataka besides niskama karma yoga and yuktahara. Training of mind, systematically, is very much necessary for transformation of consciousness. Training of mind constitutes three steps. Firstly, concept of dharana should be clear, secondly, intensity of experience and, finally, intensity of concentration. To make the second step successful, you have to practise inner visualization. But during this process, one will have to face many obstacles. They are as follows:

1. Visions – both good, like, angels, demi-gods, etc., and bad like snakes, lions, devils, etc., come up. If you are able to remain calm and unaffected, then, your practice is proceeding unimpeded.

2. Kundalini awakening – a person, in whom partial awakening of kundalini has occured, a susumna channel

has not been aroused, dharana is impossible. For this pranayama perfection is essential.

3. Sensitiveness sensual and emotional feelings develop in the lower centres, forcing you into the external world, because purification of prana and psychic centres increases the production of sexual fluid; for this, celebacy has to be maintained and sexual energy has to be transformed under the guidance of an expert master.
4. Encountering illness
5. Disillusion
6. Changing practices.
7. Applying short-cuts.
8. Excessive social activities.
9. Irregular diet.
10. Imbalanced diet.
11. Unnecessary tensions.

Once you are capable of overcoming osbstacles and you have trained your mind, you can practise the different techniques of dharana, mentioned in Yoga, Tantra and Upanisads. Some have already been discussed. The rest will be dealt with briefly, now.

The techniques are as follows, which are to be done under the guidance of an expert master.

Yogic and Tantric Dharana

1. Kaya-sthairyam - Body stability.
2. Chakra suddhi - Purification of psychic centres.
3. Ajapa-japa - Done in 10 stages.
   - one - Frontal passage rotation.
   - two - Spinal passage rotation.

- three - Frontal passage rotation with ujjayi.
- four - Spinal passage rotation with ujjayi.
- five - Arohana - avarohana rotation.
- six - Ida-pingala elliptical rotation.
- seven - Pingala-ida elliptical rotation.
- eight - Ida-pingala spinal rotation.
- nine - Pingala-ida spinal rotation.
- ten - opening the chakras.

4. Trataka - Done in 4 stages.
   - one - external concentration.
   - two - external - internal concentration.
   - three - internal concentration.
   - four - void concentration.

Upanisadic Dharana

1. External ether concentration.
2. Internal ether concentration.
3. Cerebral ether concentration.
4. Hearty ether concentration.
5. Little ether concentration.
6. Miscellaneous concentrations.
   - one - Five elements concentrations.
   - two - Chakras concentration.
   - three - Five sheaths concentration.
   - four - Five prana concentration.
7. Destructivity concentr ation.
8. The five concentration together.

□□□□

22.
MEDITATION – THE SCIENTIFIC WAY

Concentration was just fixing the mind; but meditation is allowing one idea to flow continuously. Hence, meditation is an unbroken flow of knowledge of the object on which one meditates. A person who meditates at least half an hour daily will be able to face the battle of life with peace and spiritual strength. Meditation kills all pains, suffering and sorrow. It is the most powerful mental and nervine tonic. The divine energy flows freely into an aspirant during meditation and puts up a benign, soothing influence on the mind, sense-organs and nerves. Thus, the whole body gets rejuvenated. Meditation is the key to unlock the secrets of life to open the doors of intuitive knowledge and realms to eternal bliss. For meditation, one has to cultivate burning dispassion, burning aspiration or an intense longing for self-realization. Meditation cannot be attained in a short while. One will have to struggle hard for a long time, be vigilant, diligent and persevering, with a lot of patience. All doubts are cleared on their own gradually. A mysterious inner voice will guide you. The best time for meditation is early morning, between 4 and 6 a.m.

In the beginning, the mind will need a concrete object for meditation. For that, take the form of your master or God and meditate on all the good attributes such as omnipotence, perfection, purity, freedom, absolute knowledge, etc. Later, practise meditation on abstract things like effluence of the sun, splendour of the moon, twinkle of the stars, magnificence of the ocean, with its infinite nature. Then slowly go a step forward and compare these abstract things with your own self. Finally, compare the ocean to the infinite self-consciousness-bliss-knowledge-existence, and the waves, foams and icebergs to the various names and forms of the world. Gaze on the mountains, rivers, the formless air and the all-pervading ether. This will lead you to the realization of the nameless and formless Soul. This stage of meditation is explained below :

Meditation is the state of mind, in which it is free of object-perception.

According to this settlement, dhyana means diverting the mind from worldly objects and trying to concentrate it on the self. To concentrate on the self is samadhi.

Having attained dharana, there occurs a continuous flow of perceptive knowledge of the goal of the meditation which is called meditation and in that state of samadhi the aspirant acquires the fruit of meditation and experiences his own trueself, i.e., Absolute existence–consciousness–bliss as the only reality.

Following are the possible obstacles in meditation and the process of removing them is given below:

a) **Sleep and laziness** - Eat less, keep the spine straight, increase the duration of pranayama. It is also good to have a stroll after food.

b) **Overwork and tension** – Avoid unnecessary work, share work with others, work regularly and in a planned manner and leave some things to be worked out by God.

c) **Misuse of time, things, people, etc.** – Remain careful, use everything with care and caution.

d) **Too much indulgence in pleasures** – Reflect on the uselessness of pleasures and try to become detached from them.

e) **Bad company and greed** – Best, if avoided.

f) **Basic passions** – Acting passionless and with discrimination.

g) **Tension** – Practise relaxation asanas, have good thoughts, help others without any wish, meditate for a fixed period daily at the same time, worship the Lord and visit temples.

h) **Criticising others and fault-finding** – Be forgiving and be patient with others, try to remain silent and ignore faults in others.

i) **Unhealthy body** – Practise asanas, pranayama and satkarmas.

j) **Obstacles and lack of-progress** – Have patience and balance of mind.

k) Some other obstacles are tossing of mind (viksepa), rising of latent desires, lack of celibacy, spiritual pride, diseases. For these to be overridden intensive japa-yoga, prarthana, trataka are essential. You have to destroy desires through dispassion, discrimination and study of spiritual books. Shun the company of worldly things. Practise celibacy. Give up pride and utilize all necessary means to eradicate diseases, that have come up due to past birth's actions.

l) The greatest obstacle in meditation is when the aspirant tastes the bliss of the lower stages of samadhi (contemplation) and thinks that he has attained liberation. For this, self-analysis and introspection are necessary, as this will save from such a blunder.

Following are some methods of entering into meditation which have been presented, here, keeping in mind the preliminary aspirants as well as the highest level of aspirants, i.e., adepts.

Dainandini Dhyana

At night, before going to sleep, sit in any meditative pose and, then close the eyes and concentrate on the cidakasa. Then, bring to mind all the major and important events of the day, right from the time of waking up to getting into bed. Also review your actions. Take a pledge not to repeat your mistakes and to perform right actions, even better in the future. For example, one should take a vow not to be angry, greedy, infatuated, jealous, false, deceptive, etc. Also pledge to say sorry to others for wrongs done to them and try to rectify, wrongs done by you. If necessary try to remain in silence for some time for atoning all your mistakes. This is repentation. Concentrate on good actions and be determined to remove your faults like anger, greed, etc.

Then, in the morning, after having a bath for practising the daily yoga routine, sit in some meditative pose and write down the schedule for the day in a copy, mentally. Concentrate on the order, in which the various tasks are to be done and fix a time for each. Repeat the vows taken in the previous night. During the day, perform the tasks in the decided order and in a proper manner.

You shall be very much surprised to see that in a few days you shall be able to succeed in every task undertaken and your daily routine shall be tension-free, calm and peaceful. When this happens your mind shall be better prepared for meditation.

Vigara Dhyana (Concentration on the Thoughts)

We have dealt with this topic in the chapter under the heading antarmauna. This is the second step in the process of entering into meditation. The only difference is now you are not imagining but you are only a witness of all that comes in front of you during the practice.

Breathing Speed	Element the breadth	Taste Taken	Reach of Time	Sense	Body affected	Bija affected	Mantra
Middle	Earth	Pungent	12 finger	20 secs Smell	Anal	Larh	
		breadths		opening			
Lower	Water	Sweet	16	16	Taste	Sex	Vam
Upper Fire	Bitter	4	12	Sight	Feet	Ram	
				& Navel	Touch	Hands	Yarh
Side Air	Sour	8	8				
					& Heart		
Spiral	Ether	Hot	26	4	Hearing	Mouth	Hath

Mantra Dhyana (Sylable Meditation)

This topic, too, has been covered in the chapter under the topics japa-yoga and ajapa-japa. This is the third step in the process of meditation. The only difference is now you will not be chanting even mentally but visualizing as a witness the mantra's subtle form and meditating on its resonance.

Svasa Dhyana (Concentration on Breathing)

After the first three steps, i.e., concentration on daily routine, concentration on thoughts and mantra yoga, try to concentrate on the breathing. Close the eyes and let the breathing be deep. Do not stress too much. Peacefully concentrate on the exhalation and inhalation. Remain still like a witness. Remain conscious of the pace and volume of breathing. Concentrate on the nostril, being used for breathing–the right, left or both, i.e., ida, pingala or susumna. After a few days of practice, try to notice how the breath is going in and coming out of the nostrils–from the centre of the nostril, from its lower part, upper part, right side or the left side. From the pace of breathing, one shall have to know which element–earth, water, fire, air or ether–is being transmitted. The table on previous page shall help in deciding this. Untill you have an experience of all this and you have attained control over all the methods of breathing, keep practising.

Sahaja Dhyana (Natural Meditation)

Sit in any meditative pose and close the eyes and concentrate on the breathing, as much as you can. Then, start chanting om. For some time, practise ajapa-japa. Thereafter, concentrate the inner vision on the third eye and think of your natural self. In other words, concentrate on your pacific, unified, pure divine joylike-form of true knowledge. Contemplate, thus–I am not the doer or a pleasure-seeker. Happiness-sorrow, jealousy-anger, gain-loss, victory-defeat, fame-ill fame, respect-disrespect, hot-cold and hunger-thirst all are the feelings of the mind. I am beyond all these. I am just a witness. I am the pure Brahman. I am the immortal Soul. Only, the physical body and the mind are affected by birth and death, sleep and awakened state, old age, ailments, smell, touch, beauty and words. These don't affect my true form. Hence, I am free of all boundaries of time, space and place. This is my real form. Try to concentrate the mind on such thoughts and, then, chant the mantra om and get up after chanting the shanti-patha, i.e., prayer.

Nada Dhyana (Meditation of Subtle Sound)

Literally, nada means sound or resonance. But, actually, nada means the flow of consciousness. Consciousness passes through seven states before it is perceived by the senses.

The first state is the formless, pure Brahman, which is the Divine Consciousness–the basis of the other six states of nada.

The second state is om which has three sub-forms–first is nada, second Bindu and the third kala. Nada is that state of om in which the subject and the predicate are indistinguishable nonseparate and are present in the dormant form of ignorance. This form is called saguna nirakara, a formless one, but with attributes.

In aggregate, i.e., in macrocosm, superior or universal consciousness, this form is called Tavara or God and in isolation, i.e., microcosm, individual or empirical consciousness, it is called prajna.

The third state is that of bindu. In it, subject and predicate are still indistinguishable but their form is subtle. This is called saguna sakara saksma, a subtle thing, with form and attributes. In aggregate, i.e., macrocosm, superior or universal consciousness it is called antaryami (hiranyagarbha) and in isolation, i.e., microcosm, individual or empirical consciousness, it is called taijasa.

The fourth state of ork is kala. This is the gross form of in aggregate, i.e., macrocosm, superior or universal consciousness, it is called virata and in isolation, i.e., microcosm, individual or empirical consciousness, it is called visva.

The fifth state is that of pard. It is the silent form of the sound. It is also the basic form, which is present in each person's heart, through which the mind knows the word, which is later expressed outside.

The sixth state is pagyanti. The mind "hears" it but the ears cannot. Like a dream, it is a subtle form of sound. At this stage, sound gets a mental form.

The seventh state is that of madhyama, which is obvious to the mind but not to the senses. Like the period between the state of sleep and awakeness, it lies between the gross and the subtle. It can be heard by the ear as a whispering sound but is not expressed out. Thus, by this a person gains knowledge of the meaning of the sound for himself.

The eighth state is vaikharr. It represents the words that are, spoken. This is the gross form of sound, heard by all.

Hence, the basis of nada-dhydna is the sound in the form of Brahman as stated in the ancient text *Mandukyopanisad.* In dhyana, one concentrates on the beginning of practice of nada sounds of various Indian classical musical instruments. The sounds produced from these instruments, when they are played according to classical music, activate the various chakras. Hence, in the company or under the guidance of the 'guru (master), one can gain the capability of concentrating on the sound, and thus, attain the union of the soul with the Supreme.

In the absence of a capable guru (master), one could concentrate on the music produced on a flute or a vrna. After that, one could sit in some meditative pose with closed eyes. One should shut the ears with cotton or the fingers or in some other manner so that no outside noise disturbs you. Now, one should concentrate on the inner resonance or, whatever sound, one hears within.

After practising thus, for some time, one should chant, and concentrate on the resonance, produced within, due to this chanting. Slowly, the path to the state of meditation shall open up for you.

Bhava Dhyana (Qualitative Meditation)

Sit in a meditative pose and concentrate on the cidakasa. Contemplate on the virtues of your deity, Guru or some other highly revered person in your life. Concentrate on virtues like kindness, joy, forgiveness, patience, peace, fearlessness, compassion and courage. If necessary, recall some incident or event that brought out that virtue of that person and to which you were a witness. No doubt, these virtues would be completely opposite of your own weaknesses but the thoughts of such virtues would give rise to similar virtues in you.

Bhavatita Dhyana (Transcendental Meditation)

Sit in some meditative pose for some moments with the eyes closed and remain completely silent. Be a witness and try to concentrate on the thoughts that are rising in your mind. Try to see if there are any thoughts and what they are about. Do not get involved with the thoughts. Just be a witness. Remain aware and repeat over and over again - I am not a part of the play. I am a witness. I am not the thinker. I am just a witness to my thoughts. I am the pure consciousness that is I am Brahman.

Slowly, concentrate on the sacred, pure and divine light-like Soul in between the gap between two consecutive thoughts. Chant om. With the sound of concentrate on the breathing and the prana, that is moving up and down, the susumna channel. Feel the resonance of om, all around. Feel yourself being dissipated all around in the form of divine light along with the resonance of oil. Visualize the universe present in the divine light the earth in its place in the universe your place on earth and your own physical body. Visualize yourself separate from all these as the omnipresent divine element that instills consciousness in everything. Keep concentrating on the sound of oil. When you have practised for some time, visualize the omnipresent divine element returning to the physical body. Concentrate on the divine consciousness in each part of the body and your breathing. Get up after santi-patha, the prayer.

Unmani Kriya

Sit in some meditative pose and practise five rounds of kapalabhati pranayama. Perform along with the three bandhas and then do not open the eyes. But practise ujjayi pranayama. Concentrate on the flow of pranic energy from the muladhara to the chakra and back, even as you chant om. Imagine that the sound O starts from the difla chakra and, as it reaches the muladhara, it culminates into. Repeat fifty times and, then, chant soham. Rest after every 16 chantings. Chant the soham mantra 52 times too. Again repeat with oil. Thereafter, sit peacefully for some time and experience the rise of joy and happiness within, due to the just-practised meditation. Do not fall asleep or practise for the sake of entertainment. Return to the normal state and open the eyes after santi-patha prayer.

□□□□

23.
SCIENCE OF VITAL ENERGY (PRANA–VIDYA)

We have described prana in the fourth chapter, Science of Prayanama. In brief, the divine life-force that enters the body along with the air we breathe in, is prana. Several types of prayanana have been described for achieving control over prana through the control of breathing. This is done for spiritual and physical gains. The highest science relating to prana is called prana-vidya. By practising the process being revealed, here, one can gain the capability of using, prana for the physical and spiritual good of oneself and others, too.

One can, do this practice while sitting, lying on the back or on the stomach or lying on the side. The only thing is that the spine should be straight. One should do this practice, when the right nostril is working, i.e., when the pingala channel is active. This practice is done in two steps. In the first step, while breathing in, imagine that pranic energy is flowing from the manipara chakra or each pore of the body towards chakra and accumulating there.

Then, slowly breathe out. In the second step, imagine that the accumulated pranic energy is being disseminated to all parts of the body through the various spiritual channels. Or imagine it is flowing to that part of the body where you have some pain, disease or any other part, where you want it to concentrate for special benefit. If you wish it to flow into the body of some person, use the thumb and the ring finger of the right hand to transfer the energy to the desired part of the body.

Procedure - Close the eyes lightly and become ready. Get into a comfortable position but with the spine straight and be still. Now harmonize the pace of the flow of prana with the pace of breathing.

Remember that the pranic energy moves in circles, anticlockwise. Imagine the pranic energy starting from the muladhara and moving up in a semi-circle from the right to reach the svadhisthana. Then, from there, it moves again in a semi-circle but from the left to the manipura chakra. In this manner, it rises up from one chakra to another until it reaches the chakra. Then, it returns to the muladhara from the reverse direction. This is the conscious flow of the pranic energy in wave form.

When you have become perfect in this practice, then, let the pranic energy rise, as you breathe in and, let it return, as you breathe out, normally. Also be aware of the whole process as the pranic energy rises and gets accumulated in a waveless form in the aftia chakra. Repeat in your mind that both your pranic energy and your conscious energy are getting accumulated in the ajna chakra.

After this, hold the breath in and perform the three bandhas and feel the kundalini power rising to the chakra along with the pranic energy. Relax the bandhas and breathe out. Then, let the body relax. Repeat the cycle again. Imagine that you are not breathing in and out just through the nostrils but through every pore of the body. Each time you breathe in, feel the pranic energy and the kundalini rising; and every time you breathe out, feel the body relaxing.

Then breathe in, deeply and slowly. Feel that the breath is spreading to each part of the body and the accumulated pranic energy in the chakra is being disseminated throughout the body. The pranic energy is not only flowing up and down through the chakras in the spine, but is reaching every cell of the body. The breathing should be in the form of ujjayi pranayama.

Further, imagine that you are breathing not through the nostrils or the body pores but through the chakra. With each inhalation, feel the entire body being filled with pranic energy and with each exhalation, feel the body relaxing. Feel this with a harmony between the breathing, the imagination, the inner vision, the feelings, the thoughts and the awareness of the body. Do not concentrate on just one. Feel that your body is blowing like a balloon, as all these processes go on. The body shall expand as you breathe in and relax as you breathe out. Also, there shall be dissemination of the pranic energy and relaxation of the body, respectively.

When you have mastered this practice, try to make the pranic energy flow wilfully through the various parts of the body. In the end, again, let the pranic energy disseminate with inhalation and let the body relax with exhalation. Thereafter, open the eyes. For the best use of such practices and quick progress in them, one needs the guidance of a capable guru. Do not try to do on your own. Otherwise there might be reverse results instead of benefits.

Kundalini Vidya
(Science of Kundalini – The Dormant Energy)

This is the highest form of dhyana and sadhana, i.e., meditation and spiritual practices. One should try to do this practice after getting initiation from a guru. One can practise the following practices which are being revealed here. But as the last three practices are kept secret, they are not being revealed, here. They are revealed by the guru, directly, to an eligible disciple, only.

The 19 Practices Are -

1. Viparitakarani mudra, 2. Chakranusandhana,
3. Nada saficalana, 4. Pavana saficalana,
5. Sabda saficalana, 6. Maha-mudriq,
7. Maha-bheda-mudra, 8. Mandaki kriya,
9. Tadana kriya (these practices are for masterin. pratyahara),
10. Naumukhi-mudra, 11. Sakti saficalana,
12. Sambhavi kriya, 13. Amrta-pana,
14. Chakra-bhedana, 15. Susumna dargana,
16. Pranahuti, 17. Utthana,
18. Svarapa dargana,
19. Lifiga saficalana (these practices are for mastering dharana).

After these, come the three practices, through which dhyana and samadhi are mastered.

Important Facts Related to Meditation

Some important facts relating to meditation are as follows:

1. First of all, meditation is not anything that can be forced. Just as sleep comes naturally and one cannot go to sleep by one's will, similarly, meditation happens on its own. Still one has to prepare a bed, bed cover, pillow, blanket, etc., for going to sleep. Similarly, one has to practise the above practices to prepare the mind for meditation. In fact, meditation is an experience that is beyond words just like sleep and the taste of sweets. It can be known only through experience.
2. Meditation has been described as the thoughtless state of mind, self-analysis, conscious analysis of the self, becoming still in the state of mindlessness and so on. But, actually, meditation cannot be described in words.

3. Until one has not become detached from the means of comfort in the material world one cannot dive within and meditate.
4. Actually, the mind is both a boon and a bane for humans. It is through the mind that one can become free of all bonds or get caught in the mire of this world. Hence, one has to practise meditation till order to make the mind, devoted to achieve the goal of spiritual emanciation. The ancient texts state–*mana eva karanam bandhamoksayoh.* Mind is the root cause of bondage and liberation, both.
5. Meditation is a very practical activity. There is no need for any laboratory for it. The body itself is a laboratory in which the mind and the senses are the devices. The science of turning the mind (which always tends to wander outwards) inwards and transcending it above everything can be called as meditation.
6. Through meditation only the sattva, i.e., alpha waves, the most pure among the four waves produced by the brain (alpha, beta, theta and delta, i.e., sattva, raja, tamah and migra) are generated. As a result one feels divine joy and peace.
7. The aim of meditation is to concentrate the restless mind.

Benefits of Meditation

The final aim of meditation might or might not be realization of the Soul but the following benefits surely accrue to a practitioner of meditation:

a) One gains a tension-free mind. The mind becomes still and the body relaxed and peaceful.

b) The mind is not troubled by worldly tensions because the mind, the senses and the experiences, attained through them with the divine powers, are under control of the yogi.

c) *Yogah karmasu kaugalam* – i.e., according to this verse, through meditation and Yoga, one gains the capability of performing action with wisdom as well as concentration.

d) All the chemical processes and organs of the body, start working flawlessly.

e) Problems like high blood pressure, heart ailments, mental disturbance, tension, sleeplessness, nervous disorders are cured.

□□□□

24.
CHAKRAS – THE SOURCE OF ENERGY

Everything is energy. You can facilitate the entrance of energy into your body through the top of your head. Here is one way to start learning how to consciously absorb the life force:

Sit quietly and close your eyes. Imagine warm white or blue light glowing about six inches above the top of your head. Open your head to receive the light, which flows down your legs, down your arms, and out of you. Then become filled to overflowing simply by closing your fingers and toes so the chi builds inside you. Become saturated, even to the outside of your aura, the field of energy that surrounds every organism. Become replete with energy. Take your time. Then let the light grow until it surrounds you. Notice how you feel. When you are ready open your eyes. The protection of the light will remain with you.

Chakras: Spinning Energy Wheels

For thousands of years, Eastern philosophers have believed that the human organism gets most of its energy from invisible waves or rays entering through the top of the head. Every parent knows the soft spot on a baby's head, the fontanelle, must be protected for the child's first months of life. The bones of the skull naturally close this opening with age, to protect the delicate brain tissues. Just as this opening is thought to have received energy from the mother while she holds her child in the womb,

Eastern tradition teaches that the crown of the head remains the primary entrance place of vital chi throughout life. In addition, significant amounts of chi also come up through the spine and through the feet, from Mother Earth.

As the life force enters the body, it passes through and activates the seven primary chakras. The word chakra means "wheel," and is an ancient East Indian symbol, used in this sense to mean a center of physical and psychic energy. The seven major chakras are known by many different names. We prefer the East Indian terms.

1. Muladhara
2. Svadhisthana
3. Manipura
4. Anahata
5. Vishudha
6. Ajna
7. Sahasrara

Also indicated on the accompanying chakra diagram are two secondary chakras. We like to call the palm chakra (8) by its Chinese name, Lao Kun, and we refer to the chakra in the soles of the feet (9) as Yung Chuan, " Bubbling Spring." We mention these secondary chakras in some of the dynamic meditations in Part Two, for example in Red Dragon chi kung, where pyramids are formed between the chakras .

There are, of course, many other energy points and junctions along the energy meridians (which correspond to our nervous system) which lace our bodies. The acupuncturist uses these points to cure illness and relieve pain.

The major chakras are located along the spinal column, and are closely related to the endocrine system, the nervous system, and the circulatory system, all of which influence hormonal secretions in some way. The accompanying illustration shows approximately where the chakras are located, and you can see for yourself how they relate to the diagrams of body systems.

At the peak of health and vitality, our chakras spin or vibrate at great speed. As we grow older or develop unhealthy habits and begin to lose vitality, the rate of vibration of some or all of the chakras slows down. This gradual decrease in vibration affects the flow of hormones released by the endocrine system. Too much, too little–either condition brings on the familiar symptoms of aging, and also increases the possibility of disease.

Your task is to mix and balance the incoming energy, the earth energy, with the energy coming in from the universe, and to create a system of chakras that literally "hums.". If balance occurs, each chakra will be open, the physical body will perform optimally, and a unified organism will result.

Are you "In the Pink"?

When concentrating on the different chakra centers of your body, you may see certain colours when your eyes are closed. Once your goals become more spiritual, you may feel drawn toward particular colours, depending on the chakra you are working with. It is all a matter of what feels right to you at each particular stage of your spiritual development.

Rainbow colours are almost universally accepted to represent the chakra centers, although there is not such agreement as to which colour symbolizes which chakra. But this does not point to one being right and one being wrong, rather, it points to the difference in what colour was seen by a particular master while in meditation.

The number of light waves that come to our eyes each second is known as the frequency of light. The different frequencies are perceived as different colours. The red end of the light spectrum or rainbow, is the lowest frequency of light waves. The blue end is the highest frequency.

And, of course, light is not the only thing that has a frequency because it is composed of waves of energy. All parts of the universe, flesh and blood, plant and mineral vibrate because each is a different form of energy. Our chakras are concentrations of energy which seem to have their own integrity and their own separate identity and frequency. You can "feel" someone behind you without actually hearing, seeing or noticing him or her in any way other than identifying a field of energy that is vibrating a bit differently than your energy body.

We are presenting the colour scheme and key words we are most comfortable with, based on the colours our energy work has shown us. You can adapt it according to what colours you identify with when working with each chakra.

Chakra Colours and Keywords chart I

Muladhara	Red	The base chakra relating to survival and procreation.
Svadhistana	Orange	The health and pleasure chakra relating to well being, immunity from disease and pleasure in life.
Manipura	Yellow	The power chakra or solar plexus, relating to a reservoir of spiritual and physical energy which gives strength to all the other chakras and keeps them healthy,
Anahata	Green	The heart chakra, relating to unconditional acceptance which frees the other chakras from ego, melts our heart's love energy with cosmic wisdom, and makes the bridge from physical to spiritual and from known to unknown.

Vishudha	Blue	The throat chakra, relating to creativity and self-expression, the gateway to communication with the unknown
Ajna	Violet	The third eye chakra, relating to intution, paranormal powers, and psychic awareness.
Sahasrara	Indigo	The crown chakra, relating to liberation into the cosmic realm, bliss

Develop Patience

In the West, people are competitive and impatient, attributes which do not promote spiritual development. We want to work in the stars because it sounds more interesting, more exciting; it is something new and different. English words tend to give false impressions, because of how we use the same works in everyday life. Without thinking about it, we want to rush on to do "advanced work" because it must be more important than " beginning work". And , of course, violet is a royal colour and must therefore be more deserving of our concentration than plain old red.

It is important not to make the mistake of confusing the terms "higher" and "better." Muladhara, Savadhisthana and Manipura are known as the earth-based chakras. Vishudha, Ajna, and Sahasrara are the cosmic chakra. Right now, most of us are living in the physical plane and our firm fouondation, our base, is very well developed. But the earth based chakras all need nourishment and attention. At the same time that you are developing the chakras that are symbolically higher in the body and which deal more with the spiritual aspects of life, give your three lower chakras nourishment. Even though out heads may be in the clouds, our feet are still on the ground.

The Cleansing Breath Technique

This is best done in a kneeling position in which you can bend forward freely. Place your hands on your stomach, left hand over right, just underneath your rib cage. Bend forward and gently press out all the air by pulling in with your hands and expelling all the air in your lungs.

Then, take a complete breath in about six or seven good, sized sniffs, going back each time until you are sitting upright on your heels. Your diaphragm will expand downward as your lungs fill, your stomach will push outward, and your rib cage will come up. Don't hold this large breath more than a few seconds. Release it explosively, all at once, through your nose.

Assist the rapid and complete cleansing by pulling in with your hands and by leaning forward as you exhale to get all the air out. Up to seven cleaning breaths can be done at one sitting. This cleansing breath technique is beneficial to anyone, but especially for those exposed to a polluted environment (which does include most of us).

The following technique is a breath balance which can be performed before any exercise.

Nadi Sodhana

The purpose of this "breath of union" is for you to begin to breathe equally through both nostrils. It is an effective technique for balancing the energy in your body and the two hemispheres of your brain, to help you attain a more balanced state of awareness.

To begin, sit on the floor, cross-legged if possible or in another comfortable meditation posture. Your left hand with thumb and index fingers joined rests on your left knee. The index finger of your right hand rests on your forehead, between your eyebrows at the third eye chakra. The thumb of your right hand will be used to close your right nostril and the middle finger will close your left nostril.

You will probably be breathing through one nostril more than the other. For the purpose of these instructions, we will call the right nostril the dominant one. If you find you are breathing more from the left nostril, begin the breathing sequence in reverse of what we describe, starting out with your left hand closing your nostrils, and so on.

To begin Nadi Sodhana, inhale and press your right nostril (or whichever is your dominant nostril) closed with your right thumb and exhale forcefully through your left nostril. Inhale through your left nostril as you count to seven. Now close your left nostril with your middle finger of your right hand and hold your breath again for a count of seven.

Release your right nostril and exhale through it for a count of seven. Immediately, still keeping your left nostril closed, inhale slowly through your right nostril for a count of seven. Assume Mul bandha as you make this slow inhalation. After you count to seven, close both nostrils and hold your breath for another count of seven. Now release the left nostril and exhale through your left nostril for a count of seven, releasing Mul bandha as you do so.

Repeat the entire sequence seven times in all. Remember, do not hold your breath if you have high blood pressure. You will gain a balancing benefit from this technique.

Chakra Chart II

Sanskrit	*English*	*Body root*	*Plexus and gland*
Muladhara	Root support	Coccyx, Pelvic plexus	Testes and ovaries
Swadhisthana	One's own place	Sacral vert. Navel	Hypogastric plexus
		(Below)	Adrenal glands
Manipura	Gem city	Lumbar vert. Navel (above)	Solar plexus pancreas and liver

Anahata	Unstruck Sound	Thoracic vert.	Cardiac plexus
		Heart region	Thymusgland
Vishuddha	Purity center	Cervical vert. Throat area	Pharyngeal plexus Thymus gland Parathyroids
Ajan	Command	Nasion Between eyes	Nasociliary plexus Pituitary gland
Sahasrara	1,000-petaled	Bregma Top of head	Cerebrum Pineal gland

□□□□

25.
YOGIC EXERCISES FOR RELAXATION

These exercises are very useful not only for relaxing the body but help in better sleep and mental fatigue is also removed.

Shavasna

Lie down straight with your back on the ground. Keep a distance of one foot between the legs and keeping both the hands little further from the thighs, keep the hands slightly open towards upward direction. Close the eyes, neck straight, the whole body should be relaxed. Slowly take four to five deep breaths and leave. Now, look at each part of the body through your mind with determination and experience that each organ is in relaxed condition and tension free. Determination is the force behind all the works and great objectives. Now we have to give complete rest to our body. For this also we have to take the determination of relaxing and resting the body.

First and foremost, with the determination of the mind look at the toes of legs, leave them totally loose and tension free. After toes, look at the ankles, experience their relaxation. Now see the calf muscles and think that my calf muscles are absolutely healthy, tension free and in the position of total rest and experience that the whole body is getting rest by the mere feeling of relaxation. As we start crying with the feeling of extreme sorrow, we laugh with the feeling of happiness, and the blood starts boiling with the mere feeling of victory, in the same way the body starts experiencing total rest only with the mere feeling of relaxation. After calf muscles now looking at the knees, experience that they are healthy, and in the condition of tension free. Within the mind look at the thighs and experience them to be in the condition of total rest. After thighs gradually look at the upper parts of the body–waist, stomach, back, looking at them with ease–experience the situation of total rest, health and tension free. Now with quiet feeling, concentrate the mind on the heart and try to listen to the heart beats. Listen to the divine tune of the heart and think that my heart is absolutely heatlhy, tension free and in the situation of total rest, there is no disorder or disease in my heart. Now relaxing the lungs and the heart, look at the shoulders and experience them to be in the situation of tension free and totally relaxed. Then look at hands, elbows, wrists and fingers of both the hands and big fingers and experience the hands to be in the situation of tension free, relaxed, and total rest.

Now look at the face and think there is no worry, tension, disappointment or any negative feelings on my face. There is happiness, gladness, expectation and calmness on my face. There is unlimited happiness on my face including my eyes, nose, ears. Till now we have given to give total rest to the body with the navel to give total rest to the mind and relax the mind. Now we have to move away from the thgouhts arising in the mind. For this we have to take the shelter of the soul. Think that –I am the son of the soul which is always pure-hearted, clean, pious, calm, happy, and enlighten nectar. I am always complete and immortal. I do not lack anything, in fact I am always full of feelings and devotion. I am the part of the happy form of the God. I am the nectar son of the God. I am separate from the bonds of nature, body, senses and mind. My natural shelter is my God. I do not become pauper, poor, orphan or possessing a parent or guardian or a king with the increase and decrease of outside prosperity. I am always one essence. The changes which are taking place are the duties of the world, my soul has no duties. In this way think about the divinity of the soul and remove the negative thinking, because negative thinking makes a person sad, worried, and stressed. Negative thinking makes a person depressed and always immersed in the ocean of grief. Positive thinking person is always happy, normal, and cheerful even in the adverse situations. For this reason, the person should have positive thinking not only at the time of yoganidra or shavasan but during the whole day. In this way we have thought positive about the divine form of the soul and gave rest to the mind and now we will think about the divine form of the God and give total rest to our soul.

Think that your soul has come out of the body and it is lying above the body in the sky and you are experiencing with the internal soul that the body is lying on the ground just like a dead body. This is the reason that this asana is called Shavasan. Now devote your conscious strength to the God who is spread in the unending sky in the form of Supreme Soul–Brahma. Think that your soul is the divine happiness of the God from all sides. Experience the divine happiness of the God's creation. The determination which is auspicious and with completed devotion towards God, is complete. You think of this God's nature and its divinity and concentrating on the wonderful form and creation of nature think of God's divinity. Think that you are in the valley of beautiful flowers, and the whole atmosphere is full of the scent of the different kinds of beautiful flowers. There is a kind of divinity on all sides. It is a great sight to see the God's creation. There is no end to God's creation. Along with the flowers, plants, there are beautiful fruits on the different trees, the God has filled each fruit with different flavors. A light breeze is flowing from all sides and giving immense happiness. In this beautiful garden the birds are chirping, the divine songs of the God's creation. One can see God appearing from each flower, fruit. When we look at the sky it appears that the stars, the Moon and the Sun are like diyas in the huge universe in the form of temple. The rivers are flowing as if they are washing the feet of the God. Brahma is so great, unlimited, unbounded, unending. Oh God ! Oh Father ! Creation of the earth, Oh Mother ! Take your son also in your shelter. Bless me with your divine happiness. Oh Lord ! I should always get your divinity, calmness and enlgihtment. I should always remember your divine creation and immerse in you, and be engrossed in the unending happiness. Oh God ! take me out of the wordly feelings and take me in the lap of happiness.

In this way take the incomparable happiness and once again experience yourself in the body. Imagine that you have returned back to the body after full sleep of Yoga. The respiration is on. Along with the breath the great power of life source is entering inside you. Experience yourself to be healthy, happy and cheerful and in the way the body was relaxed with determination in the same way and with the same determination experience the new power, co sciousness and happiness in the body. Look at each organ from toe to the head and whichever organ you are seeing imagine that it is absolutely healthy. For example, if a person has pain in the knee or backache he should imagine that his pain has been relieved. By God's grace and practice of Yoga there is no pain in my knees and back, because Yoga cures the root cause of these diseases. The pain is coming out. In the same way there is any heart or stomach problem think that it has been cured. If there is any blockage in the arteries and the cholesterol level is high then think that the diseases are being cured. Take the vow that all the foreign particles, diseases, and deformities are going out and I am totally healthy. With these thoughts you should experience yourself to be physically and mentally healthy.

In the end experience that both the hands are totally powerful and healthy and rub both the palms against each other and keep the warm palms on your eyes and slowly open the eyes. This is the summarized method of Yoganidra and Shavasan. If anybody is unable to sleep then before going to bed, practice Shavasan and relax the body and feel tension free in the directed method and think of God's divinity and concentrate on the respiration and with every breath chant Omkar in the mind. While inhaling and exhaling meaningful chanting of Omkar should be done. The meaning of Omkar is Brahma in the form of God, Omkar God is always in the form of truth, consciousness and cheerful. I am also getting happiness by praying the Omkar God. With these thoughts one should chant Omkar. The speed of inhaling and exhaling should be normal. In the same process count reverse from 100 to I and with each number chant Om. For example Om 100, Om 99, Om 98 etc. Praying in this way will put you off to deep sleep and you will get rid of bad dreams. In the daily yoga practice, this asana should be done after every difficult asana. After the end of practice, this asana should be done for 5 to 10 minutes.

Benefits:

1. Mental stress, depression, high blood pressure, heart disease and insomnia are cured. These patients should do this asana regularly.
2. Weakness of the nervous system, tiredness, negative thinking are cured.
3. The body, mind, brain and soul gets total rest, power, zeal and happiness.
4. The concentration power increases.
5. Practicing Shavasan in between asanas relieves the tiredness of the body.

Makarasana

Process:

1. Lie straight with your stomach towards the ground. While folding both the hands keep them on the opposite shoulders.

2. Rest the forehead on the hands. There should be one foot distance between the legs.
3. Relax the body like a dead body. While lying down in this position think of a dead body and concentrate yourself within the soul through wise thinking and introspection. I am a separate life, pure-hearted and cheerful and flawless soul. This body is perishable. This body is the collection of five elements. When the time comes it merges in the same elements. This body and other riches remain here. We do not bring anything with us neither we will take anything along. In this way deviate your mind from the mortal world and experience the happiness of devotion to the Brahma present in the unending universe.

Benefits:

1. This is the asana for rest. During rest a person feels light not only physically but also mentally. He is free from high blood pressure, mental tension and insomnia. In-between the asana this should be done for rest. The intestines of the stomach get natural massage which activates them and dysentery and other deformities are cured.
2. Since the hands are in passive stretching condition it affects the sympathetic nerves and helps in the relaxation of the body.
3. The heart does not function against the magnetic force, therefore it gets rest.
4. The internal secretion glands are benefited.

Balasna (rest position)

Process:

1. Lie down with your stomach towards the ground. Keep the left hand under the head on the ground and turning the neck to the right keep the head on the hands, the left hand

will be under the head and the left palm will be under the right hand.

2. Fold the right knee slightly, the way a child sleeps, lie down like that and rest. In the same way this asana is done from the other side.

Benefits:

Just like Shavasan, the tiredness of the body and mind is relieved.

26.
DIET FOR THE YOGA PRACTITIONERS

A well balanced diet contains sufficient quality of protein, carbohydrates, fats, salts and minerals. It is said in Reiki that "as you eat, so you become". This is because the kind and quality of food affects the physical as well as mental conditions of the individual. In Yoga all foods have been divided into three categories–Rajasi (Royal), Tamasi (Carnal) and Satvik (Noble). The Rajasi food comprises a variety of dishes. This type of food includes fried, roasted and fatty stuff, which is not desirable for good health. A little intake of these types should be sufficient to titillate the palate. A little quantity of strongly spiced bitter or sour food (Tamasik) should also form part of diet which should mostly be made easily digestible, nourishing; and freshly prepared food which classifies the noble or Satvik food. Your food must give you the variety of all the six varieties of taste–sweet, salty, astringent, bitter, sour and biting. However, it is not only the quantity or quality of the food but your way of eating which is also very important. Whatever food you eat, masticate it thoroughly and allow the saliva to reduce the eaten morsel to a mere pop before gulping it down. Always eat 75 to 80% of your total capacity and leave enough room for the movement of gas/liquid etc. to help the system digest the eaten food quickly. Drinking water with food should be totally forgotten. Drink water always half an hour before and half an hour after your having food. Drink enough of water between your meals but not with it.

For your help we are giving below some guidelines following which you shall remain healthy. Adherence to them will not only keep diseases and disorders at bay but enhance also the age of your healthy life.

- The food that we eat helps build the blood cells, nerves, bones and muscles in our body. It has been proved scientifically that food which is highly processed and high in protein, fat, salt and sugar leads to health problems. Nutritious food (balanced wholesome diet, moderate exercises, drinking enough water, that is 8/10 glasses (3 litres) of water, enjoying fresh air and sunshine, resting adequately every day, will ensure a healthy body and mind.
- Detoxify the system completely by fasting 2 to 4 days every three months with liquids, preferably fresh lemon water with honey 4-5 times daily and follow it up with an all fruit course for 5 to 7 days and then resort to normal diet cautiously and gradually. Take enema on the days of fasting immediately after taking mud pack for 15/20 minutes. Also take abdominal pack at night.
- Abdomen must be kept cool and soft always. All liquid intake should be close to the body temperature as far as possible. Take mud pack, hip bath, enema and oil massage intermittently.
- Drink 1 or 2 glasses of water on rising, every morning.
- Dental health plays a vital role in curing a troubled abdomen. An unhealthy abdomen; an unhealthy abdomen is responsible for most of the dieseases.
- Use honey and molasses instead of sugar. Use a lot of garlic and some ginger if they suit. Take maximum roughage/fibre.

- Avoid non-vegetarian, concentrated, stimulating, intoxicating and gas forming foods.
- Ideal time for lunch is 10.00 a.m. and for dinner 7.00 p.m. May take some fruits (one variety only) around 2.00 p.m. Take only two meals a day and satisfy 80% of your hunger or appetite. Do not eat if not hungry or in bad mood/anger or at odd hours.
- Shun smoking, tea, coffee, alcohol, zarda, pan-masala, soft drinks and drugs.
- Going for brisk walk and/or doing Yoga for 30 to 60 minutes daily is a must.
- Wash vegetables and fruits properly under running water, scrubbing with a brush before cutting, as they contain pesticides and contaminates. If any germs are suspected then wash in water with diluted solution of potassium permanganate.
- Ensure good digestion, sound sleep, good appetite and evacuation of bladder and bowels regularly and naturally.
- Tension is very harmful, as it causes flatuence, constipation, irritability, besides liver and heart problems. Hence change the way of living. Do not work for long hours. Do Shavasana and enjoy minimum 7 hours sound sleep daily.
- Always use polyunsaturated oil and reduce salt and sugar intake to the minimum possible level.
- After lunch, rest a while and after dinner, walk a mile–is a wise old recommendation. Relax in Vajrasana for 10-15 minutes afte the meal.
- Take very light but nutritious food which includes fruits, skimmed milk and yoghurt (curd).
- For healthy condition, 80 percent of alkaline foods to 20 percent alkaline diet is needed. Alkaline food and drink

purify the bloo . Refined and processed foods tend to acidify and pollute the blood and the cells.

- Select your food from the following.

a) Acid producing foods

All fresh foods, fish, pulses, white bread, polished rice, white flour, nuts, confectionery, sweets, coffee, tea, alcohol, boiled buffalo milk, fried foods, concentrated foods, hydrogenated stuff, beans, onions peanuts, tomatoes, jam and all preservatives, pickles, unripe fruits, refined stuff, grapes and high protein foods.

b) Alkali producing foods

All kinds of vegetables, potatoes, fresh fruits, butter milk, fresh lemon, coconuts, figs, dates, almonds, loquates, skimmed milk,yoghurt, molasses, sweet oranges, dry fruits, sprouts, whole flour/unpolished rice and honey.

Foods to be replaced/limited

- Limit intake of cheese and red-meats that are high in saturated fat content.
- Number of calories, obtained from fat, must be kept below 30% of total daily dietary intake of calories.
- Not more than 10% of total fat calories should be obtained from saturated fat intake.
- Avoid processed and junk foods that are overloaded with flavouring preservatives and colourings.
- Butter should be replaced with soft margarine or low fat foods that are high in polyunsaturated fats. Spread it thinly.
- To keep the blood sugar level within normal confines, consume sugar in limited quantity.
- Salt intake must be limited. Avoid eating salty foods, and also adding (extra) salt to meals. Also do not consume processed meats and crispy eatables.

- Limit use of tea, coffee, cold drinks, chocolates and sweets so as to reduce intake of caffeine. Instead you may use herbal teas with advantage but without hassles.
- Excessive intake of alcohol must be reduced.
- Do not use strong spices and condiments as they irritate stomach.

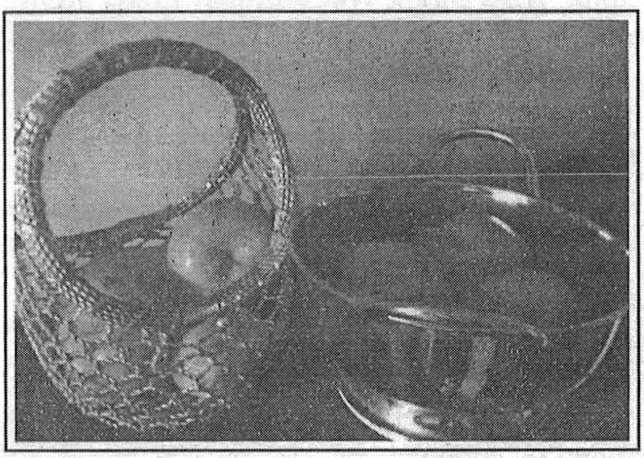

Ideal Menu and Timings

- On rising early in the morning, drink a glass or two of normal water.
- Take a glass of juice (carrot/apple with sweet lime/ orange) before going for a brisk walk around 7.00 a.m. (during summer 6.00 a.m.) May take a cup of skimmed milk after vigorous yogic exercises, if suits.
- Lunch (10:00 a.m.)

  Take nutritious food as you need

  Take good Salad (consume first),

  enough energy for working whole

  cooked vegetables 2 or 3 cups, medium day

  chapati 2-3 or rice 2 cups, 2 cups

cooked pulse , 1 or 2 cups of youghurt
(Dahi), steamed vegetables 1/2 or 1 cup.

- Supper (Around 7:00) p.m.)

Out of total 1600 Calories consumed
As per your taste and chioce but
during the whole day, evening meal
light, e.g. (A) 1 or 2 cooked veg
should not contain more than 350
vegetable, with 1 chapati, and 1 calories
cup of yoghurt or (B) 1 cup soup,

1. fruit and raw vegetables or (C)
2. cups of skimmed milk with 1 or 2 bananas or apples or toast or bread slices.

- If you have to go out for dinner, take just a cup of skimmed milk or soup or eat some roasted grams or some fruits/ vegetables at around 6:00 p.m. before going. If you take a late evening dinner, drink a glass of lemon juice (juice of 1 lemon in one glass of warm water) the following morning (empty stomach).

Herbs And Spices

- You may use asafoetida (Hing), cloves, corriander, garlic, ginger, saunf, turmeric, cumin (jeera), cardamon, ajwain, pepper, and kali rai.
- Bed tea/coffee is very harmful. Avoid tea/ coffee/cold drinks and fried items always.

□□□□

27.
NATURE'S TONIC
–DRINK WATER IN EARLY MORNING

Water is panacea for chronic and incurable diseases. Rise early from bed. Do not wash your face and mouth as you do normally. Sit comfortably and drink four large glasses of water. Do not take any thing for 45 minutes. You can wash your face and brush your mouth after drinking water.

Always drink water after an hour of breakfast and meals. If sick persons or soft natured persons with a delicate physique are unable to take four glasses of water at a stretch, they should start from one or two glasses and then gradually they should start taking four glasses. Take four glasses of water regularly. Experiments have proved that different diseases can be cured within the time given below by its regular use:

Hypertension	-	Within one month
Gastric trouble	-	Within ten days
Cancer	-	Within six months
Constipation	-	Within ten days
Diabetes	-	Within one month
TB	-	Within three months
Leucorrhoea	-	Within one month
Paralysis	-	Within three months

Other diseases described above may be cured within four to six months according to their nature. Drinking four glasses of water does not have any ill-effects on health. Only urge to pass urine will be great and you will pass urine in large quantities frequently. Passing of stool will be easy and complete. It will facilitate the expulsion of the accumulated waste matter very effectively and leave you fresh.

Besides hydrotherapy certain other measures or household remedies are also advised for such disorders.

Role of Water on Stomach

There is secretion of stomachic juice in stomach to digest food. The more genuine the stomachic juice, the better digestion of food.

If someone takes liquid whether it is water, wine or beer, the stomachic juice will not remain genuine. It would be adulterated by the intake of water, wine or beer and would not be effective in digestion of food.

Similarly, if some person takes water six or eight times while taking his meal, it would liquidate stomachic juice so much that it would not be able to act as digestive juice.

Do not take water at all during meals. If you have to take it, take very small quantity of it, so that genuine stomachic juice may be absorbed in all eaten food.

If you feel thirsty after one hour or more of taking food, please take water in limited quantity. Body especially stomach needs water at interval from time to time to liquidate its juice, to increase its quantity and to absorb the solid material (food). The body itself informs whenever it needs it. Sometimes, the desire to take water is slow and sometimes it is very fast. One should be particular about intake whether it is from healthy or sick stomach. One should take it as much as it is sufficient and good for health.

It should be taken at equal intervals of time especially when one is suffering from fever. One should not take a glass of water at a stretch but each five or ten minutes in less quantity. Intake of water at a stretch by a patient of fever, will not quench his thirst, rather it would increase other symptoms of illness.

Water taken in less quantity is at once accepted and absorbed by stomach. Repetition of its intake at each half-an-hour produces juice in more quantity and removes whole dullness and constipation by flowing in body and intestines. It cools them also.

One can use luke warm water or cold water according to its taste.

Use of Water

1. Saline water is necessary in dehydration caused by cholera, fever, diabetes, diarrhoea, etc.
2. It is useful to take water with salt, sugar, lemon and honey. Patients of kidney diseases should use water with salt in supervision of some naturopath.
3. Some of vegetables, water of pulse, sharbet of lemon and juice etc. contain water. They give us minerals and salts along with water.

Regular intake of water in early morning gives relief in following diseases:

1. Diabetes
2. Acne, Boils
3. Headache
4. Blood pressure
5. Old age and wrinkles
6. Arthritis
7. Paralysis problem of ladies
8. Anaemia
9. Heart diseases, Faintness
10. Cold, Cough, Asthma, Bronchitis
11. Obesity
12. Meningitis
13. Disorders of liver
14. Tuberculosis

15. Disorders of the eye
16. Irregular menstruation
17. Urinary problems, Stones, etc.
18. Hyperacidity Asthma, Bronchitis
19. Gastric trouble and diseases concerned with back, Spine
21. Swelling, Fever
20. Cancer of ovary
22. Digestive disorders
23. Piles
24. Diseases caused by Vata, Pitta, Cough.
25. Mental weakness, etc.

Some Important Facts

1. Never drink water before passing urine or just after passing urine.
2. Passing urine after meals prevents formation of stones.
3. Stand on forefoot and then pass urine. This posture prevents formation of stones.
4. Water contained in copper vessel is hundred times more useful.
5. Take juice of one lemon in a glass of warm water before going to bed. It gives relief in Coryza.
6. Take juice of one lemon and teaspoon of honey in warm water in morning. It helps in curing obesity and improves complexion.
7. In early morning, chew five leaves of Neem (Azadiracta indica) and Holy Tulsi (Ocimum basilium) and drink a glass of water after chewing these leaves. This can prevent you from carcinoma (Cancer) and plague too.
8. Take a little rice (raw-one or two teaspoons) with a glass of water to cure liver disorders.
9. The water kept in a Shankh for a whole night is remedy for stammering speech. Continue this for four to six months.

28.
TIPS WITH YOGA

While you are practising Yoga, you should also ensure that your lifestyle is such which keeps your energy body clean, positive and strong. This will be very favourable to your Reiki healing practices.

1. Stop or minimize caffeine drinks (e.g. coffee, tea, soft drinks, chocolate etc.). They create imbalance in the nervous and endocrine system and hence in the energy body.
2. Stop alcohol intake.
3. Minimize taking sweets and white sugar products.
4. Stop or minimize smoking.
5. Refrain from eating meat, such foods contain lot of toxins secreted by animal during killing. Moreover, meat is considered Tamsik food with lot of negative energy.
6. Do occasional fasting with water and fruit juices. It will keep your system clean.
7. Relax and meditate regularly. Sitting postures of meditation (with straight spine) help a lot for balancing your pranic flow in the body.
8. Reduce time in watching TV, listening to radio, reading newspapers and stray magazines. Excessive involvement in

these things distract the mind and thereby affect the balance of energy body.

9. Go for regular walks in morning/evening in fresh air. Do moderate exercises and yogasanas with special emphasis on spinal exercises to keep it supple and straight.
10. Drink water stored in gold, silver or copper vessels. Water charged with these metals becomes filled with positive energy. Magnetized water is equally good.
11. Do pranayama or breathing exercises. They are very effective in balancing and strengthening your energy field. Specially develop the habit of rhythmic and diaphragmatic breathing as your moment to moment resting breathing. It has a very benevolent effect in maintaining a healthy aura.
12. Spend time with nature whenever you get apportunity. Take sunbath in the morning. Fire element of our body is easily rejuvenated by sunbath.
13. Have regular water bath and do friction rubbing of body either by hand or by bath brush before bathing. Bathing in flowing river water is very good. Occasional bathing with salt water helps in cleasing the negative energy as salt has the charactersitic of breaking down the negative energy. Among salts, sea salt is said to be especially useful.

    Some people do foot soaking in salt water. Water can be lukewarm, hot or cold depending upon your body's demand at a particular time. This is a very effective method for removing the negative energy of the body through the feet which is sucked by salt water. After foot soaking, this water should be thrown into W.C. because this water becomes impure after absorbing negativity.

    Foot soaking in salt water is said to clear our Swadhisthana and solar plexus chakra.

14. Walk barefoot on earth specially near river and countryside and on grass wet with morning dew. The earth element sucks lot of negativity through our feet and clear our Mooladhara chakra (or Root chakra). Sole chakra is an extension of Root chakra and is related directly to it. Sole chakra is also said to be related to Heart chakra.
15. Increase your awareness and attention in every task you do. This will increase your power and sensitivity to sense subtle impressions and sensations within and around you.
16. Laugh a lot. Laughing is a potent medicine for supplying you with instant positive energy. If you find difficult to laugh in your normal life routine, then read jokes in magazines/books, see comedy serials on TV, read entertainment columns of magazines etc. Also develop the habit of cutting and hearing jokes frequently (within limits of decency). Try to wear a natural smile on your face. This will keep you effortessly positive.
17. Be aware of negative emotions (e.g. anger, fear, jealousy, hate, worry, impatience, hurry, revenge, etc.). Whenever they are arising in you, nip them in the bud at the very outset. Negative emotions throw your energy body completely out of balance
18. Take some measures for keeping your home and work environment clean for creating a positives energy field as mentioned below:
    i) Evaporate pure camphor crystals. An easy way to do it is with the help of an electronic mosquito repellent. Place the camphor on a used mat. This way the camphor evaporates very slowly over many hours.
    ii) Burn incense ('agarbatti's and 'dhoops'). Their smell also purifies the energy of the surroundings.

iii) Following oils have the power to create positive energy and neutralize negative energy. Hence burn oil lamp of the following oild:

a) Mustard oil

b) Sesame (Til) oil

c) Ghee or clarified butter

iv) Candle burning also neutralizes negative energy and creates positive energy. 'Trataka' on candle flame is very good because its light clears out the negative energy. This practice is said to clear Ajna Chakra.

v) Salt water specially sea-salt water has great potential for neutralizing negative energy. One can mop the floor with sea-salt water or one can even keep a bowl of sea-salt water in a corner of the room. Every now and then put the bowl in the sun for a few hours and top it up and also change the water completely after certain days.

vi) Fresh cut flowers with leaves and stems intact, placed in water in a vase or bowl and indoor plants are great positive energy generators and negative energy neutralizers. Yellow, orange and blue/violet flowers are quite good for this purpose.

vii) Use those colours in your surroundings (room walls, curtains, carpet, furniture, wearing clothes) which promote positive energy and transmute negative energy. Such colours are white, blue, violet, green, yellow, orange, rose etc. Even visualizing these colours in meditation helps you in getting their positive energy.

viii) Just like colours, there are certain sounds which generate positive energy and transmute negative energy. All satwik sounds and music come under this category. These sounds are found generally in old melodious songs and music, devotional songs, sould stirring bhajans, classical music, flute music, sound vibrations generated by blowing into a conch shell ('shankh') and sounds simulating nature sounds e.g. sound of waterfall, flowing river, moving breeze, chirping of birds etc. By listening to such sounds, you always feel calm, centred, joyful and elevated. On the other hand, the modern Rajasik music like pop music only gives momentary thrill and excitement and hence it is not good for energy body.

ix) Foodgrains, specially rice (uncooked), have the capacity to absorb and transmute negative energies. In particular, on the eleventh day of the waxing and waning moon cycle, this absorption is at a maximum. This day is called 'Ekadasi' (eleventh day). Hence they are kept in 'Pooja' (worship) places.

x) Tulsi leaves are very effective in destroying the negative energy and purifying the atmosphere by creating positive energy. Hence always keep Tulsi plants in your terrace/balcony.

xi) Chanting of Mantras and Nam-Japas creates an energy pure environment mainly because of effect of pure sound vibrations. However, mental japa of mantras is equally effective in purifying the environment because the pure thought vibrations created by mental japa also act on the energy atmosphere around because of the relationship between thought and life energy.

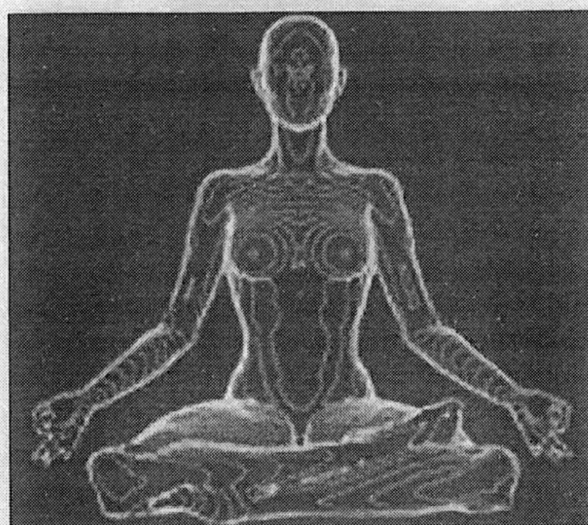

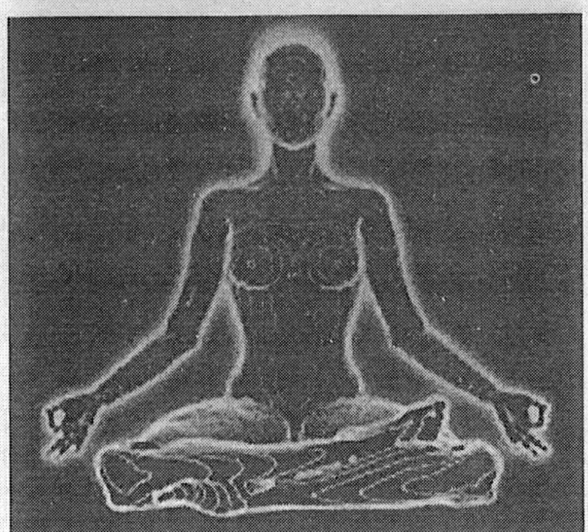

THE EIGHT LIMBS OF YOGA

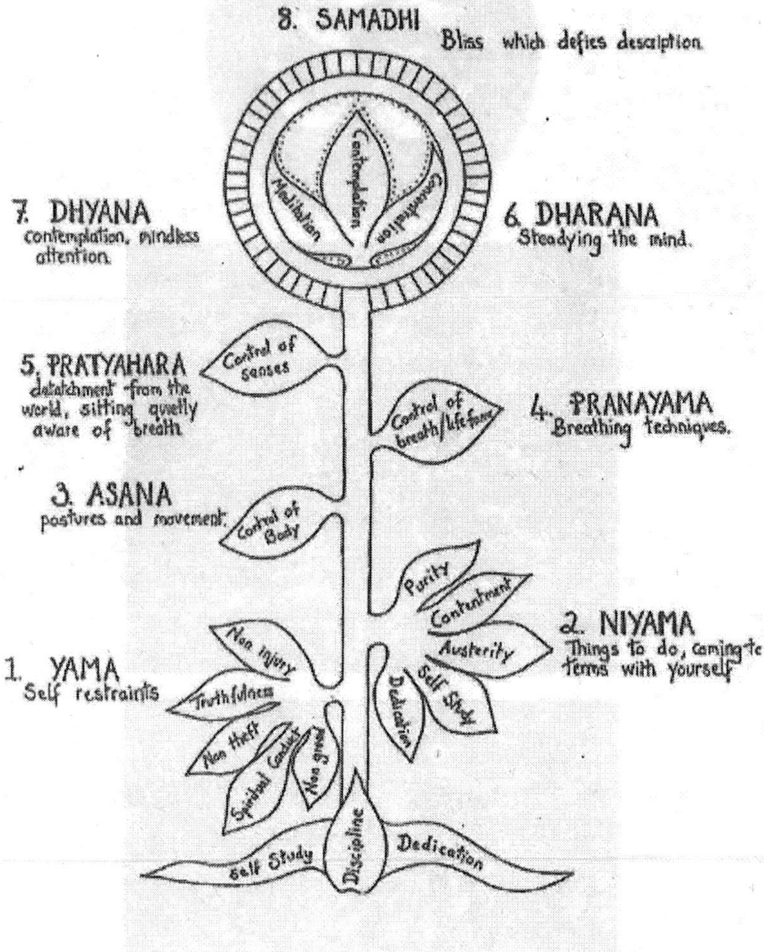

25. Sex Education
26. Common Diseases and Cure
27. Pranayama for Better Life
28. Herbal Home Remedies
29. A Guide to Beauty & Skin Care
30. A Guide to Heart Care
31. A Guide to High Blood Pressure
32. Cancer: Causes and Prevention
33. Child Care and Nutrition
34. Nature Cure for Common Diseases
35. Good Health Through Food and Regimen
36. A Guide to Allergies
37. A Guide to Aging
38. Ayurveda for Health & Beauty

Lotus PRESS